DRUG DOSAGE IN LABORATORY ANIMALS
A HANDBOOK

DRUG DOSAGE
in
LABORATORY ANIMALS
A HANDBOOK

by C. D. BARNES
and L. G. ELTHERINGTON

Revised and enlarged edition

University of California Press — Berkeley, Los Angeles, London

UNIVERSITY OF CALIFORNIA PRESS

BERKELEY AND LOS ANGELES, CALIFORNIA

UNIVERSITY OF CALIFORNIA PRESS, LTD., LONDON, ENGLAND

© 1964, 1973 BY THE REGENTS OF THE UNIVERSITY OF CALIFORNIA

ISBN: 0-520-02273-4

LIBRARY OF CONGRESS CATALOG CARD NUMBER: 64-21066

2ND REVISED AND ENLARGED EDITION, 1973

3 4 5 6 7 8 9 0

PREFACE TO THE FIRST EDITION

This handbook was conceived as a result of the authors' frustration in attempting to find appropriate drug dosage for use in laboratory animals. The few available sources of information were limited in the number of species or the routes of administration. This handbook is designed to provide a concise and up-to-date reference source of available drug dosage in seven commonly used species of laboratory animals. Parenteral and oral routes of administration are included.

We are grateful to the following individuals and firms for dosage information made available for use in this book.

DR. R. M. FEATHERSTONE, CHAIRMAN,

DEPARTMENT OF PHARMACOLOGY, UNIVERSITY OF CALIFORNIA, SAN FRANCISCO MEDICAL CENTER

DR. J. J. BOSLEY, STANFORD	HOFFMAN-LA ROCHE, INC.
RESEARCH INSTITUTE	LAKESIDE LABORATORIES, INC.
DR. B. GRAHAM, STANFORD	MERCK INSTITUTE
RESEARCH INSTITUTE	RIKER LABORATORIES, INC.
ABBOTT LABORATORIES	SANDOZ PHARMACEUTICALS
BURROUGHS WELLCOME & CO.	SCHERING CORPORATION
(U.S.A.), INC.	SMITH, KLINE AND FRENCH LABORATORIES
CHAS. PFIZER AND CO., INC.	THE SQUIBB INSTITUTE
CIBA PHARMACEUTICAL COMPANY	THE UPJOHN COMPANY
ELI LILLY AND COMPANY	WYETH LABORATORIES

Our special thanks go to Mrs. Joan Sauer and Miss Tina Moya for their assistance in the preparation of the manuscript.

PREFACE TO

THE REVISED EDITION

The first edition of this handbook was favorably accepted and appeared
to fill a "need" of many investigators. There were, however, two major
criticisms concerning "a lot of blank spaces" and omission of "favorite
drugs." There is no question that, somewhere in the published literature,
drug dosage information exists which would fill some of the blank spaces.
We have simply not found this information. In our judgment, the value of
the book, which contains over 4600 doses and 1278 references, far out-
weighs this justifiable criticism. We deliberately designed the format so
that an investigator could add special interest drug and dosage information to his own "personalized" handbook. The selection of drugs included
or omitted from this handbook was governed by two considerations: first,
our judgment as to general interest in the drug and second, our finding
enough information about the drug to justify its inclusion.

We have expanded this second edition to include 9 new drugs, 459
additional references and more than 1050 new doses. The sections on
factors modifying drug response and anesthesia have also been expanded
and brought up to date, as has the appendix listing physiological solutions.

CONTENTS

INTRODUCTION

This handbook provides pharmacodynamic and toxicologic dosage for drugs commonly used in biomedical research. The primary consideration governing drug selection was to include typical representatives of major drug groups. Chemotherapeutic agents were omitted because animal dose information is available from the package inserts which accompany veterinary preparations. A secondary selection criterion was the reported use of a drug in several animal species and via more than one route of administration. Some research compounds and drugs with a specific or limited spectrum of use (for example, radiation-protective drugs) were deliberately omitted because they do not satisfy this requirement. A number of new drugs that show promise of future widespread use clinically, or as experimental tools, are included even though they do not yet meet the specified criterion.

Drug responses are classified according to (1) toxicity, (2) primary use or action, and (3) secondary uses or actions. To present effeciently as many doses as possible, it was sometimes necessary to classify a number of specific drug actions and uses under one general heading. For example, a cardiovascular category may include drug effects on cardiac output, regional blood flow, vascular resistance, mean arterial blood pressure, etc. A behavior classification may represent drug-induced alterations of conditioning, learning, sociological behavior and spontaneous motor activity. Where available space and sufficient information permits, single drug effects or uses are listed separately. Since the dosage entries are referenced, the technique of grouping drug effects and uses allows tabulation of more doses in a limited space, thus reducing the handbook size without sacrificing completeness. Toxicological data are included to provide information relating to the upper part of a drug dose-response curve thereby assisting the investigator in choosing a maximally effective dose

1

that produces minimal toxicity. In some instances lethal doses were obtained for an animal species or route of administration for which no pharmacodynamic information was found. Lethal doses are presented in the following order of importance: (1) LD_{50}—lethal dose 50%, the dose, calculated statistically, sufficient to kill 50 per cent of the population; (2) MLD—minimum lethal dose, the dose reported sufficient to kill a single member of an experimental group; and (3) LD-lethal dose, the dose which has been reported to kill an unspecified number of an experimental group.

Drugs are listed in alphabetical order according to the nomenclature suggested by the World Health Organization (WHO) drug dictionary, as published in World Neurology, September, 1961, or the Merck Index. Wherever possible, three common and/or trade names are included and cross-indexed with the official name. All in vivo doses are expressed as milligrams per kilogram of body weight (mg/kg) of the "commonly used" salt.

The introductory material, discussing factors modifying drug response and anesthesia, is a simplified presentation of basic pharmacological and rational anesthetic principles necessary for maximum data validity in acute animal experiments. Biomedical research literature contains much contradictory information which may be partially explained by differences in anesthetic agents or techniques and indifference to basic pharmacological principles in the design and interpretation of experiments.

Table I contains a list of injectable anesthetics commonly used in seven species of laboratory animals. For reasons discussed in the previous section, these "fixed," injectable anesthetics are recommended only for chronic or recovery experiments. Inhalation agents are suggested as the only rational means of providing general anesthesia for acute, non-recovery experiments.

Appendix A presents hormone maintenance and replacement doses which have been reported to be effective following surgical removal of endocrine glands. The material is referenced, and tabulated under the surgical name of the animal following gland removal, e.g., hypophysectomized.

In vitro concentrations, expressed as milligrams per 100 ml of bathing solution (mg%), are included for use of investigators studying drug effects on isolated organs or tissue. The information is presented in a tabular form and space has been allowed for addition of new concentrations and responses of particular interest to the investigator. Similar to the in vivo material, all concentrations refer to the "commonly used" salt. Non-referenced concentrations are from laboratory teaching experiments, familiar to the authors, in which the bathing or perfusing solution was aerated with 95% oxygen and 5% carbon dioxide and maintained at 37° C.

A recent publication (1157) provided valuable information on classical techniques for studying isolated preparations.

FACTORS MODIFYING DRUG RESPONSES

Rational drug administration to laboratory animals involves two major considerations: (1) pharmacological action, i.e., influence of the drug on the animal and (2) drug disposition, i.e., influence of the animal's "milieu interieur" upon uptake, distribution and elimination of the drug. The tabular portion of this handbook provides dosage information related to pharmacological action and this introduction will briefly consider physiological and pharmacological factors which influence drug disposition.

PHYSIOLOGICAL FACTORS

Age. A young animal, especially newborn, exhibits differences from the adult in drug absorption, metabolism, excretion and sensitivity. For example, hepatic enzyme systems responsible for the biotransformation of barbiturates are deficient in the newborn (1245) resulting in increased drug sensitivity. Nonmetabolized drugs may produce a greater effect because of decreased renal function or increased access to receptor sites, for example, greater blood-brain barrier permeability.

Endocrine. Any major hormonal imbalance may be expected to influence drug action. Adrenal insufficiency attenuates the vascular effect of catecholamines and hypothyroidism enhances the respiratory depression of narcotic analgesics. Animals that exhibit circadian rhythms, such as

3

the mouse, may demonstrate marked differences in drug response related to the day-night time of administration (1246).

Health. Animals used for drug studies, especially those who are to receive general anesthesia, should be in the laboratory environment at least two weeks prior to the experiment. Observation of dietary habits, character of stool and general physical status should exclude "sick" animals. A procedure for the preoperative evaluation of dogs (1247) could be modified and applied to the pre-experimental preparation of any laboratory animal.

Nutrition. A starved animal with depleted glycogen stores exhibits a much greater sensitivity to cardiovascular and central nervous system drugs. Likewise dehydration, with subsequent hypovolemia and altered volume of drug distribution, may result in enhanced drug toxicity.

Sex. Drug disposition differences between males and females of some species (especially rats) are probably related to hormonal differences. For example, in male rats barbiturate sleeping times may be increased by administration of female sex hormones to equal those of the female (1248).

Species. Quantitative and even qualitative differences in drug disposition have been shown to exist between species and even within different strains of the same species. They are apparently related to different rates and/or pathways of drug biotransformation. For example, the dog is unable to metabolize codeine to morphine and rapidly demethylates ephedrine, whereas the rat excretes part of the administered codeine as morphine and hydroxylates ephedrine as the primary inactivating pathway (1249, 1250).

Temperature. The influence of body temperature on drug effects may be subtle and unknown or quite striking (1251). Mild hypothermia in the dog (32-33° C) results in a 30 per cent decrease of metabolism while moderate temperature decline (28-30° C) elicits a 50 per cent decrease

4

in metabolism, heart rate and blood flow (1252). Hyperthermia produces an elevation of metabolic rate and cardiac output. Changes in body temperature, easily monitored by rectal or esophageal thermometer, may result from: (1) heat loss secondary to anesthesia-induced vasodilation, (2) heat gain from a warm environment, drug effects and excessive draping, (3) tracheal cannulation and subsequent loss, especially in the dog, of a considerable part of its heat-regulating system.

Temperament. Drug disposition in the conscious animal will be markedly influenced by the animal's reaction to handling and manipulation. Variations in the duration and intensity of auditory, visual and musculo-cutaneous stimulation will result in central-nervous-system-induced cardiovascular changes that may alter drug disposition. The use of trained animals will reduce but not eliminate these variations. Likewise, a struggling, frightened animal requires a larger dose of anesthetic agent for induction which, particularly with the use of "fixed" injectable agents, may result in a drug overdose.

PHARMACOLOGICAL FACTORS

An excellent comprehensive discussion of the many pharmacological factors which influence drug disposition may be found in a recent textbook (1253). A factor of great importance apparent from any consideration of drug disposition is drug interaction. The following discussion of the pharmacological factors important in the uptake, distribution and elimination of drugs will attempt to provide examples of drug interactions that influence drug disposition.

Route of Administration.
Drugs may be administered enterally, or parenterally. The former involves the gastrointestinal (G.I.) tract and hence the oral, sublingual and rectal route, while the latter bypasses the G.I. tract and refers to all other routes. Route of administration is important in consideration of speed of onset, intensity, and duration of drug action.

ORAL ADMINISTRATION (PO)

The oral route of administration in animals is often used for the study
of chronic drug effects or to determine factors relating to efficiency of
gastrointestinal absorption. For acute experiments, this route frequently
results in slow or unpredictable absorption of the drug and is seldom
used except in industrial screening. In some animal species (mouse,
guinea pig, rat, and rabbit), the passage of a stomach tube is relatively
easy. Other species (cat, dog, and monkey) react violently to attempts at
intubation.

PARENTERAL ADMINISTRATION

<u>Intravenous (IV)</u>. This route is often preferred for administering com-
pounds in solution. Its primary advantage is that the investigator is able
to slowly titrate the amount of drug needed (determined roughly by con-
sidering the animal's weight, age, sex, etc.) to elicit a particular response.
Also, some drugs which are tissue irritants can be safely administered
intravenously. For this technique, sharp needles and clean syringes are
very important. The skin over the vein should be shaved and, if possible,
pulled taut to prevent the vein from moving. Application of small amounts
of a rubefacient such as xylene will elicit vasodilation and facilitate injection. The skin and vein should be pierced in separate thrusts of the needle
to avoid running the needle through the vein and producing a subsequent
hematoma. A practical disadvantage of IV injection in cats, dogs, and
monkeys is that usually two persons are required for the procedure.

<u>Intraperitoneal (IP)</u>. This method of injection is one of the most popu-
lar means of administering nonirritating chemicals. The peritoneum of the
abdominal cavity presents a large absorptive area, and as long as the
needle is placed in the midline below the umbilicus and directed approxi-
mately 45° cephalad, there is little danger of piercing the abdominal
viscera. This technique may usually be performed by one person, even
with cats and dogs, but provides a relatively slow onset of drug effect

compared to IV injection. Two major problems are associated with the method. One is the "single shot" dose used; since it is not possible to titrate the drug, an overdose may be administered to a sensitive animal. Secondly, most of the absorbed material enters the portal circulation and there may be significant hepatic inactivation of the compound before reaching its site(s) of action. Another consideration with the intraperitoneal route is the volume of fluid injected. Volume is especially important in small animals such as mice, rats, and guinea pigs, and can produce volume effects which may be manifested as physiologic changes unrelated to the pharmacologic properties of the drug being studied. There is evidence that even the concentration of the solution used may considerably alter experimental results, e.g., LD_{50}.

Intramuscular (IM). A drug may be given intramuscularly in an aqueous solution, an aqueous suspension, or in a solution or suspension in oil. The drugs are administered directly into the muscle where they spread out along the muscle fibers and fasciae. This distribution affords a large absorbing surface and results in gradual absorption. The IM route of administration is particularly useful when a prolonged effect is desired.

Subcutaneous (SC). The subcutaneous route is used only for administering non-irritating drugs. This technique may result in a slow absorption of some drugs, especially vasoconstrictor agents. Compounds which cause local vasodilation, such as some local anesthetics, often incorporate a vasoconstrictor to slow down absorption. The site of SC injection may be quite important. For example, drugs which are administered to elicit an action on thecentral nervous system and are metabolized by liver enzymes should be injected into subcutaneous areas which do not drain into the portal circulation. A common site of SC injection is the back of the neck. In this area there is usually ample loose skin which can be raised, eliminating the possibility of an intradermal injection. Aspiration of the syringe before injection will assure that the needle is not lying in a blood vessel. A modification of SC administration is pellet implantation under the skin of the back (for example, desoxycorticosterone acetate).

Intrathoracic (IT). Injection of drugs high in the seventh intercostal space is a route of administration second in rapidity of onset only to the IV method; it is used extensively in veterinary medicine. There are objections to this route of administration due to the possibility of irritating lungs and pleura, but such irritation is probably insignificant in acute experiments. The amount injected should be less than that used by routes other than IV.

Drug Absorption

The two major factors affecting the amount and rate of drug absorption are:
A. Drug Factors
   1. Charge and lipid solubility
   2. Concentration gradient
   3. Geometry and functional grouping
   4. Molecular size
   5. Particle size and physical state
   6. Solubility and rate of dissolution
B. Barrier Factors
   1. Absorbing surface area
   2. Bowel activity
   3. Enzymatic activity
   4. Stomach emptying time
   5. pH of the compartment
   6. Vascularity and blood flow of the compartment

Membrane (barrier) permeabilities (for example, gut to blood, blood to urine and urine to blood) depend upon the transport process, whether it is passive, as in the case of diffusion and filtration, or active. Most drugs are salts of weak acids or bases and are passively transported across membranes based upon the pH-partition hypothesis—i.e., only lipid-soluble, unionized molecules can move down a concentration gradient. The stomach has a low pH and consequently weak acids, such as the barbiturates, exist primarily in the unionized state and are absorbed at a rate dependent upon their lipid solubility. However the narcotic analgesics, such as morphine, are weak bases and absorbed poorly from the stomach. Drug interactions can markedly influence absorption; for example, epinephrine produces vasoconstriction thus delaying the absorption of local anesthetics; narcotic and sedative-hypnotic drugs produce respiratory depression and delay the uptake of inhalation anesthetics; alkalosis will decrease the amount of phenobarbital entering the brain and increase the amount excreted in the urine.

Protein Binding.   Many drugs are bound to plasma proteins, especially albumin. Only the free drug in the plasma can pass to receptor sites and elicit a pharmacological effect. Any attempt to describe intensity of drug action in terms of blood level will be frustrated, unless the degree of protein binding is known and by the fact that the percentage of bound drug varies with plasma concentration. Competitive protein binding has been demonstrated between muscle relaxants and local anesthetics (1254) and a large number of other drugs (1253). A knowledge of protein binding is mandatory for the investigator who is studying drug-receptor interactions by the use of agonist-antagonist drug combinations.

Distribution.   Once a drug enters the circulation a constant distribution and redistribution occurs until it is finally eliminated from the body. Blood flow, protein binding and the blood-tissue partition ratio initially determines drug distribution to receptor, storage (fat, bone, etc.) and biotransformation-excretion sites. This is followed by redistribution of the drug from primary receptor and storage sites to secondary and/or biotransformation-excretion sites. The short duration of thiopental anesthesia is due to a combination of metabolism and redistribution of the drug from brain to muscle and fat (1255). Changes in the distribution of cardiac output, such as in shock, would shunt blood from liver, muscle and fat and produce higher plasma and hence brain levels, resulting in a more intense and longer lasting anesthetic state. Renal and/or liver disease would likewise alter drug disposition and result in intensified drug action.

Biotransformation.   The term detoxification was formerly used to describe drug metabolism but was discarded when it became apparent that

9

some drugs are metabolically <u>activated</u> in the body. For example, the antidepressant activity of imipramine is mediated by its metabolite desmethylimipramine (1256). Most drug biotransformation occurs in liver microsomes and involves microsomal enzyme, cytochrome p-450, reduced nicotinamide adenine dinucleotide (NADPH) and molecular oxygen. This system is reviewed in several excellent papers (1253, 1257, 1258). Only brief generalizations will be presented here. Acceleration of drug metabolism or "enzyme induction" has been demonstrated in animals following the repeated administration of barbiturates, analgesics, tranquilizers, antihistamines, sex hormones, oral antidiabetic drugs, anti-inflammatory agents and many others (1259). While prior drug exposure may be controlled by the investigator to some extent, the fact that insecticides, herbicides and various other hydrocarbon compounds are capable of inducing enzyme synthesis or possibly blocking enzyme activity creates a potential source of variation in drug disposition between and within animal species. For example, narcotic analgesics, diethyl ether, chloramphenicol and antidepressant drugs have been shown to inhibit hepatic enzymes (1259). Use of chloramphenicol as a laboratory antibiotic prolongs barbiturate sleep in dogs and cats (1260).

<u>Excretion.</u> Most drug elimination occurs via the kidney except in the case of inhalation agents and a few compounds that are excreted into the bile. Even the metabolic products of some of the halogenated inhalation anesthetics are excreted in the urine (1261) and their metabolism can be "induced" by other drugs. They in turn have the ability to "induce" enzymes responsible for metabolizing other drugs such as phenobarbital (1262).

Factors which govern drug absorption and distribution also play a role in determining urinary excretion. Since reabsorption of weak acids and bases from the urine also depends upon the pH-Partition Hypothesis, urine acidification will facilitate clearance of amphetamine and ephedrine while favoring reabsorption of barbiturates and salicylates. Respiratory acidosis, secondary to hypoventilation in spontaneously breathing anesthetized animals, or respiratory alkalosis produced by mechanical hyperventalation, may have profound effects on the absorption, distribution and excretion of some drugs.

An increasing number of investigators are using drugs in experimental animals, some in only a "minor" way (for anesthesia) and others for purposes of pharmacological investigation. This introductory material is designed to provide a general background for understanding the many variables that interact to govern the magnitude, onset and duration of drug action. The following section, on anesthetic principles and techniques, will emphasize factors governing the uptake, distribution and elimination of anesthetic agents.

ANESTHESIA

Anesthetic principles and techniques used in biomedical research have been recently reviewed (1263). Unfortunately, the review fails to distinguish the marked differences between the anesthetic technique for acute (non-recovery) experiments and that for chronic (recovery) experiments. The two experimental conditions require vastly different techniques and anesthetic considerations. General anesthesia may be produced by injection of "fixed" drugs such as barbiturates, chlorolose, urethan, etc.; or by inhalation of "variable" agents such as the anesthetic gases, nitrous oxide and cyclopropane or the volatile hydrocarbons diethyl ether, fluroxene, forane, halothane and methoxyflurane. Principles of drug disposition, discussed in the introduction, especially apply to the "fixed" agents since there is a continuous distribution, redistribution, metabolism and excretion of, for example, pentobarbital, and this results in a continual change in brain concentration and hence anesthetic state. For chronic experiments, a changing state of anesthesia presents no problem providing overdose is avoided and analgesia and immobility are maintained. Similarly, "fixed" agents for preanesthetic medication or use as adjuncts to general anesthesia may be rationally used in recovery experiments but these same drugs, as well as "fixed" general anesthetic agents, provide a varying intensity of drug effect as a background for collection of experimental data. Interpretation of data derived from acute experiments using barbiturate type anesthesia is subject to great difficulty because of the animal's constantly changing homeostatic background. The description of barbiturate anesthesia as "an abnormal physiologic situation" (1264) should perhaps be applied to the use of any "fixed" anesthetic. The popularity of α-chloralose for cardiovascular and neurophysiological studies is based upon the drug's apparent lack of reflex and cardiovascular depression compared to the barbiturates. In one study of left ventricular dynamics following a small single dose of chloralose (60 mg/kg, IV), it was demonstrated that the heart rate, bloodpressure and cardiac output of dogs did not change from awake values over a three-hour period (1265). However, when attempts were made to keep a constant "level" of anesthesia by infusion of chloralose (330 mg/kg, IV) over a three-hour period, there were marked fluctuations in cardiovascular parameters (1266). Unfortunately, any attempt to maintain a constant brain concentration of "fixed" anesthetic by means of I.V. infusion and using some "sign of anesthesia level" such as depression of corneal pain or other reflexes is doomed to result in wide fluctuations of the anesthetic state. In a study of five injectable anesthetics, using I.V. infusion and a variety of "signs of anesthesia," it was found that only walking and freedom from ataxia appeared in the same order with all drugs tested and furthermore, a sign of "deep anesthesia" such as depression of the patella reflex often persisted until the animal was capable of spontaneous movement (1267). To further diminish the possibility of achieving a constant anesthetic state, the same author showed that acute tolerance occurs—during a single exposure to the five injectable anesthetics studied the central nervous system appears to adapt to the presence of the drug (1268). This means that even assuming a constant brain concentration could be maintained (a very difficult task when one considers the many dynamic factors we have discussed which affect drug disposition) the anesthetic "level" will change with time.

Inhalation anesthesia and the avoidance of "fixed" preanesthetic drugs appears to offer the closest approximation to a constant anesthetic state for acute experiments. In chronic experiments where data is collected under anesthesia several times, anesthetic stability via inhalation agents is mandatory. The uptake and distribution of inhalation anesthetics has been recently reviewed (1269). The great advantage of inhalation compared to injection anesthesia is that once equilibrium has been established, alveolar, arterial and brain concentrations are equal. Therefore, monitoring

12

alveolar (end-tidal) concentration, and maintaining it constant by altering inspired concentration, assures a constant brain concentration and hence anesthetic "level" except for one problem. A recent study (1270) showed that cardiovascular adaptation in man occurs over a five-hour period of anesthesia with cyclopropane, diethyl ether, fluroxene and halothane. Perhaps this reflects an acute tolerance similar to that seen with the injection anesthetics (1268). However, the same study reported unpublished observations that no time-related cardiovascular adaptation occurs with halothane in the dog. These observations would have to be extended to other animal species before one could be certain that laboratory animals do not show acute tolerance to inhalation anesthetics. A recent publication from the same laboratory (1270) reported that no circulatory adaptation occurs in man anesthetized with forane, a new folatile hydrocarbon anesthetic that is not metabolized in the body.

The concept of minimum alveolar concentration (MAC), i.e., the alveolar concentration of inhalation agent required to prevent gross muscular movement in response to a painful stimulus, was introduced in 1963 (1271). MAC has been determined in a number of laboratory animals, most recently the rat (1272), and provides a technique for maintaining a constant "level" of inhalation anesthesia within and between experiments, thus markedly reducing the variability of experimental data which has been traditionally obtained on a constantly changing anesthetic background.

Utilization of the MAC technique for acute experiments in laboratory animals involves expensive apparatus for dispensing and monitoring inhalation agents but in our opinion this expense, when compared to that of other "routine" laboratory supplies such as polygraphs, stimulators, oscilloscopes, etc. is justified on the basis of more precise control over anesthesia and subsequent greater validity of collected data. A reflection of this view is demonstrated in a neurophysiological study (1273) where the authors state that inhalation anesthesia more approximates a "normal" brain state, produced by an encéphale isolé preparation, than do animals underbarbiturate anesthesia.

It is well to note that morbidity and mortality, in animals that must recover from anesthesia, is much greater following fixed agents, especially pentobarbital, than following inhalation agents. This is probably due to the long recovery time, accompanied by heat loss, pneumonia, etc., aggravated by lack of post-operative care.

No matter whether an inhalation or fixed general anesthetic is chosen, there is a good possibility that the agent will add unknown variables to the experiment. Perhaps the most outstanding example of anesthesia interfering with experimental results concerned the initial investigations of the sensory pathways between peripheral receptors and the cerebral cortex. Under anesthesia, the pathways seemed to be quite simple, but recent research has shown that while primary pathways for afferent stimuli, such as those in the thalamus, are unaffected by deep anesthesia, the secondary reticular pathways are depressed. Another example of anesthetic interference is a report by Gutman and Chainovitz (815). Small doses of pentobarbital, light anesthesia with ether or nitrous oxide, or injection of morphine converted blood pressure responses to painful stimuli in the rabbit from pressor to depressor. Chlorpromazine, an anesthetic adjunct, attenuated the reaction but did not convert it. The authors also mentioned that the same induced reversal of blood pressure response occurred when stimulating the mesencephalic reticular formation. Finally, Page and McCubbin (809) concluded from their experiments that the greatly augmented depressor activity of ganglionic blocking agents in dogs following pentobarbital anesthesia probably depends upon nearly complete inhibition of parasympathetic, cardioinhibitory activity and partial suppresion of sympathetic compensatory reflexes by the action of pentobarbital. The above examples serve to demonstrate the problems which may arise from using anesthetic or anesthetic adjuncts which modify the physiological parameters under investigation.

The final part of this section provides suggestions regarding the use of general anesthesia in acute animal experiments. Seemingly insignificant or self-evident procedures are included, as these are often overlooked by an investigator:

Blood volume. Measurement of central venous pressure (CVP) and urine output will allow infusion of salt solutions to replace losses from bleeding, tissue trauma and other causes of dehydration.

Empty stomach. Animals should be fasted for at least twelve hours prior to administration of the anesthetic as a safeguard against the possibility of vomiting during the experiment and the subsequent aspiration of the material into the lungs.

Rapport. "Making friends" with the animal will contribute much to a smooth anesthetic induction. Attempting to anesthetize a frightened, struggling animal, often made that way by undue restraint, may lead to fatal consequences due to the use of more anesthetic than normally required.

Route of administration. Injectable anesthetics should be administered intravenously whenever possible. This allows titration of a maximally effective dose. Intrathoracic, subcutaneous, and intraperitoneal injections may also be utilized for administration of fixed anesthetics but possess the disadvantage that a single-dose injection may be lethal to a sensitive animal.

Temperature maintenance. Whenever possible, the esophageal or rectal temperature of anesthetized animals should be monitored. If the temperature is known, a heating pad can be used as required to maintain a constant body temperature.

Unobstructed airway. Placing a tracheal cannula or endotracheal tube in an anesthetized animal provides a patent airway and permits aspiration of accumulated secretions which might impair respiratory exchange.

Ventilation. All general anesthetics and many of the drugs used for preanesthetic medication and during anesthesia are respiratory depressants. Adequate ventilation cannot be assessed by "extent of chest wall expansion and the persistence of bright red arterial blood" as has been reported. Only measurement of end-tidal or arterial carbon dioxide tension ($PaCO_2$) and maintenance within a normal range assures adequate ventilation. Hypoxemia with resultant metabolic acidosis can be avoided with certainty only by measuring and correcting any deficits in arterial oxygen tension (PaO_2) and pH. Acid-base changes can profoundly change the disposition

15

of both injected and inhalation drugs by altering ionization, receptor sensitivity, tissue perfusion, metabolic and excretory mechanisms, etc. A sophisticated review of anesthesia and ventilation is presented in a recent publication (1277).

ANESTHETIC DOSES

The following pages present a list of fixed anesthetics and preanesthetic medications which have been successfully used in various animal species. In some instances two or more agents are listed to be used in combination. For example, atropine, morphine, and pentobarbital have been used in combination to produce anesthesia in a dog. In this case, the atropine and morphine are administered 30 and 29 minutes, respectively, prior to the pentobarbital. These two premedication agents serve to reduce the incidence of parasympathetic secretions and provide analgesia prior to administering the pentobarbital. Following the tables is a list of the major advantages and disadvantages associated with some of the more widely used anesthetic agents.

TABLE 1

Anesthetic Doses

Species	Anesthetic[a]	Page[b]	Time[c] (min.)	Route[a]	Dose (mg/kg)	Reference
Mouse	Amobarbital	40		IV	54	65
	Barbital	52		IV	234	65
	Chloral Hydrate	69		IP	400	LM[d]
	α-Chloralose	70		IP	114	204
	Chloretone (in 50% alcohol)			IP	175	LM
	Hexobarbital	118		IV	47	392
	Pentobarbital	181		IV	35	111
	Phenobarbital	193		IV	134	65
	Probarbital	210		IP	75	66
	Secobarbital	238		IV	30	63
	Thiopental	260		IV	25	111
	Tribromoethanol	266		IV	120	66
Rat	Amobarbital	40		IV	55	63
	Barbital	52		IP	190	125
	Chloral Hydrate	69		IP	300	197
	α-Chloralose	70		IP	55	205
	Diallybarbituric Acid	86		SC	60	66
	Hexobarbital	118		IP	75	393
	Pentobarbital	181		IV	25	111
	{ Pentobarbital			IP	35 }	1164
	{ Chloral Hydrate			IP	160 }	
	Phenobarbital	193		IV	100	589
	Probarbital	210		SC	225	66
	Secobarbital	238		IV	17.5	63
	Thiopental	260		IV	25	111
	Tribromoethanol	266		IP	550	547
	Urethane	272		IP	780	127
Guinea Pig	Amobarbital	40		IV	50	63
	Chloral Hydrate	69		IP	400	1164
	Chloretone (in 50% alcohol)			IP	175	LM
	Pentobarbital	181		IV	30	111
	{ Pentobarbital			IP	35 }	1164
	{ Chloral Hydrate			IP	160 }	
	Phenobarbital	193		IP	100	LM
	Secobarbital	238		IV	20	63
	Thiopental	260		IV	20	111
	Tribromoethanol	266		IV	100	66
	Urethane	272		IP	1500	LM
Rabbit	Amobarbital	40		IV	40	72
	Barbital	52		IV	175	LM
	α-Chloralose	70		IV	120	LM
	{ Morphine		30	SC	10 }	LM
	{ Chloretone (in 50% alcohol)			PO	175 }	
	Diallylbarbituric Acid	86		IV	50	LM

[a]Other routes of administration may be found in the main body of the handbook.

[b]The page numbers refer to the main body of the handbook where additional dosage information may be obtained.

[c]The numbers refer to time elapsed (in minutes) before the injection of the following drug.

[d]LM means that the dose was obtained from a pharmacology teaching manual.

TABLE 1 (continued)

Species	Anesthetic	Page	Time (min.)	Route	Dose (mg/kg)	Reference
Rabbit (cont'd)	Hexobarbital	118		IV	25	LM
	Paraldehyde	179		IV	300	7
	Pentobarbital	181		IV	30	111
	Phenobarbital	193		IV	200	590
	Probarbital	210		IP	66	66
	Secobarbital	238		IV	22.5	72
	Thiopental	260		IV	20	111
	Tribromoethanol	266		IV	80	66
	Urethane	272		IV	1000	LM
	{ Urethane			IP	700 }	305
	{ Pentobarbital			IP	40 }	
Cat	Amobarbital	40		IV	11	24
	Barbital	52		IV	200	LM
	Chloral Hydrate	69		PO	250	LM
	α-Chloralose	70		IV	75	208
	{ α-Chloralose			IV	50 }	747
	{ Urethane			IV	50 }	
	{ α-Chloralose			IV	80 }	748
	{ Pentobarbital			IV	12 }	
	{ α-Chloralose			IV	80 }	154
	{ Pentobarbital			IV	6 }	
	Diallylbarbituric Acid	86		IV	36	291
	Hexobarbital	118		IV	25	66
	Paraldehyde	179		IV	300	7
	Pentobarbital	181		IV	25	111
	Phenobarbital	193		IP	180	LM
	Secobarbital	238		IV	25	63
	Thiopental	260		IV	28	24
	Tribromoethanol	266		IV	100	557
	Urethane	272		IV	1250	LM
	{ Urethane			IP	400 }	749
	{ α-Chloralose			IP	50 }	
	{ Urethane			IP	280 }	750
	{ Diallylbarbituric Acid			IP	70 }	
	{ Urethane			IP	360 }	408
	{ Diallylbarbituric Acid			IP	90 }	
	{ Urethane			IP	250 }	LM
	{ Pentobarbital			IP	30 }	
Dog	Amobarbital	40		IV	50	LM
	Barbital	52		IV	220	LM
	{ Barbital			IV	250 }	LM
	{ Thiopental			IV	15 }	
	{ Barbital			IV	220 }	422
	{ Pentobarbital			IV	15 }	
	Chloral Hydrate	69		IV	125	LM
	α-Chloralose	70		IV	100	209
	{ Morphine		30	SC	1 }	490
	{ α-Chloralose			IV	100 }	
	{ Morphine		60	SC	1 }	753
	{ α-Chloralose			IV	80 }	

TABLE 1 (continued)

Species	Anesthetic	Page	Time (min.)	Route	Dose (mg/kg)	Reference
Dog (cont'd)	α-Chloralose			IV	50	LM
	Thiopental			IV	15	
	Morphine		30	SC	10	LM
	Chloretone (in 50% alcohol)			PO	225	
	Morphine			SC	1	966
	Thiopental			IV	20	
	Hexobarbital	118		IV	30	66
	Paraldehyde	179		IV	300	7
	Pentobarbital	181		IP	30	497
	Drip—6 mg/kg/min.			IV		
	Morphine		30	SC	10	751
	Pentobarbital			IV	20	
	Morphine		30	IM	2	747
	Pentobarbital			IV	15	
	Morphine		60	IM	3	458
	Pentobarbital			IV	12	
	Atropine		30	SC	1	
	Morphine		30	SC	10	LM
	Pentobarbital			IV	30	
	Phenobarbital	193		IV	80	591
	Phenobarbital			IV	200	LM
	Thiopental			IV	15	
	Secobarbital	238		PO	40	63
	Thiopental	260		IV	25	716
	Tribromoethanol	266		IV	125	557
	Urethane	272		IV	1000	413
	Urethane			IV	480	752
	α-Chloralose			IV	48	
	Morphine			IV	2	
	Morphine		60	SC	2	742
	Urethane			IV	250	
	α-Chloralose			IV	60	
	Morphine		60	SC	3	LM
	Urethane			IV	50	
	α-Chloralose			IV	13	
	Diallylbarbituric Acid			IV	8	
	Morphine		30	SC	5	LM
	Urethane			PO	1500	
Monkey	Amobarbital	40		IV	40	63
	Pentobarbital	181		IV	25	111
	Phenobarbital	193		IP	100	161
	Secobarbital	238		IV	17.5	63

TABLE 2

Advantages and Disadvantages for Anesthetic Agents and Adjuncts

Agent	Advantages	Disadvantages
1. Injection Anesthetics	Inexpensive, easy to use, rapid onset.	Constantly changing anesthetic state. Poor reproducability.
α-Chloralose	Less reflex depression than barbiturates. Catecholamine release may support circulation (1266).	Low water solubility. Inject warm or in a 10% solution with propylene glycol 200.
Pentobarbital	Rapid onset. High water solubility.	Marked cardiovascular and reflex depression.
Thiopental	Short duration (15-30 min.). Useful to induce anesthesia prior to inhalation agents.	Solution rapidly decomposes. Remains in the body a long time (1255).
Urethane	Little reflex depression. High water solubility. Long duration.	Liver and bone marrow toxicity. Used only in acute experiments.
Dial (Ciba)*	More rapid onset and less toxic than urethane alone. Less reflex depression than with barbiturate alone.	Urethane toxicity limits use to acute experiment.
2. Inhalation Anesthetics	Constant and reproducible anesthesia, therefore less data variability.	More skill required. Expensive equipment. Alveolar tension difficult to monitor in animal smaller than rat. (1272).
Cyclopropane	Rapid induction. Easy to measure—as difference from oxygen (1274).	Explosive, circulatory adaptation. Tendency to laryngospasm.
Diethyl Ether	Respiratory stimulation. Good muscle relaxation.	Explosive and stimulates secretions. Long duration in body fat. Circulatory adaptation occurs.
Fluoroxene	Cardiovascular stimulation. Little respiratory depression.	Irritating and explosive over 4%. Circulatory adaptation. Metabolized in the body.
Forane	No metabolism. Non-explosive. No circulatory adaptation ---> "constant" anesthetic state.	New drug (1970). Expensive. Cardio-respiratory depression.
Halothane	Rapid induction. Non-explosive and potent.	Expensive. Cardiovascular depression and adaptation. Sensitization of myocardium to catecholamines.
Nitrous Oxide	Not metabolized. Easily measured (1275) and used (1278).	Only analgesia in safe concentrations. Need muscle relaxants to prevent movement.
Methoxyflurane	Potent and non-explosive. Non irritating to respiratory tract.	Alveolar-arterial gradient. High fat solubility -----> long duration in body. High oxygen flows to vaporize.

*Contains: Urethane, 400 mg/ml.
Diallylbarbituric Acid, 100 mg/ml.

TABLE 2 (continued)

Agent	Advantages	Disadvantages
3. Adjuncts to <u>Anesthesia</u>	Facilitate induction and maintenence of anesthesia.	"Fixed" drugs and not advised for acute expirements.
Atropine	Decreases tracheal secretion and vagal bradycardia.	Ganglionic blockade and CNS effects.
Phenothazine (Chlorpromazine)	Preanesthetic sedation.	Many pharmacological actions, especially çardiovascular depression.
Curare	Immobility with minimal anesthesia or with nitrous oxide. "Ordinary doses" do not enter brain (1276).	Release histamine. Need artificial ventilation.
Succinylcholine	Rapid onset and short duration. Can titrate I.V. Immobility with minimal anesthesia.	Increased serum K^+. Implicated in malignant hyperthermia. Other cholinergic actions.
Narcotics (Morphine)	Analgesia and sedation facilitate anesthesia. Use as only anesthetic if support ventilation.	Release histamine. Respiratory depression causing delay in induction of inhalation anesthesia.

DRUG DOSAGE TABLES

ACETALDEHYDE
(Ethanal, Acetic Aldehyde, Ethylaldehyde)

mg/kg		Mouse	Rat	Guinea Pig	Rabbit	Cat	Dog	Monkey	
Lethal Dose $Y-LD_{50}$ $Z-MLD$	IV				Y300 [3]	300 [4]			
	IP		500 [2]						
	IM								
	SC	Y560 [1]	Y640 [1]		Y1200 [3]				
	PO		Y1900						
Hypnotic	IV						8.5 [4]		
	IP				700 [4]				
	IM				700 [4]				
	SC				700 [4]				
	PO								
Sympatho- mimetic	IV					10 [5]	10		
	IP								
	IM								
	SC								
	PO								
	IV								
	IP								
	IM								
	SC								
	PO								

IN VITRO

mg %	Cardiac	Vascular	Gut	Uterine	Visceral	Skeletal		

ACETANILIDE

(N-phenylacetamide, Antifebrin, Acetylaniline)

mg/kg		Mouse	Rat	Guinea Pig	Rabbit	Cat	Dog	Monkey	
Lethal Dose $Y-LD_{50}$ $Z-MLD$	IV					13.5 [11]	300 [11]	300 [7]	
	IP	Y820 [946]	Y800						
	IM								
	SC	1300 [6]							
	PO	1840 [7]	Y800 [8]	1500 [7]	1500 [11]	250 [11]	700 [12]		
Toxic Dose	IV						62 [7]	275 [7]	
	IP								
	IM								
	SC	1200 [7]							
	PO	1840 [7]	500 [10]		1200 [7]		700 [7]	600 [7]	
Analgetic Antipyretic	IV								
	IP	110 [946]	400 [9]						
	IM								
	SC								
	PO					*125	*500		
	IV								
	IP								
	IM								
	SC								
	PO								

*Total dose

IN VITRO

mg %	Cardiac	Vascular	Gut	Uterine	Visceral	Skeletal		

ACETYLCHOLINE

(Acecoline, Arterocoline, Ovisot)

mg/kg		Mouse	Rat	Guinea Pig	Rabbit	Cat	Dog	Monkey	
Lethal Dose Y—LD$_{50}$ Z—MLD	IV	Y20 [13]	Y22 [13]		Y0.3				
	IP	Y>125 [904]							
	IM								
	SC	Y170 [13]	Y250			Y10 [15]			
	PO	Y3000 [13]	Y2500 [13]						
Parasympatho-mimetic	IV	0.004 [1197]	0.002 [855]		0.01	0.01	0.01		
	IP								
	IM								
	SC				1.0 [14]				
	PO				1,000 [14]				
Nicotinic (Atropinized Animal)	IV				0.1	0.1	0.1		
	IP								
	IM								
	SC								
	PO								
	IV								
	IP								
	IM								
	SC								
	PO								

IN VITRO

mg %	Cardiac	Vascular	Gut	Uterine	Visceral	Skeletal	Trachea	
Guinea Pig	0.025		0.01	0.02	0.02 [16]		0.04 [1157]	
Rabbit	0.003 [16]		0.02 [16]	0.05 [16]	0.07 [16]			
Dog			0.003 [16]	0.1 [16]	0.03 [16]			
Rat			0.0002 [1157]	0.01 [1157]		1.0 [1157]		

ACETYLSALICYLIC ACID

(Aspirin, Acetophen, Acesal)

mg/kg		Mouse	Rat	Guinea Pig	Rabbit	Cat	Dog	Monkey	
Lethal Dose $Y-LD_{50}$ $Z-MLD$	IV				Z700 [4]				
	IP	Y495 [17]	Y500 [19]						
	IM								
	SC				Z700 [23]				
	PO	Y1100 [18]	Y1500 [20]		Y1800 [18]		Y3000		
Analgetic Antipyretic	IV								
	IP	25 [908]		269 [22]					
	IM								
	SC	22 [908]	20 [948]						
	PO	100 [908]	450 [21]	300 [923]	*500 [4]	*200 [24]	*200 [24]	100 [25]	
Toxic Dose (Convulsant)	IV								
	IP								
	IM								
	SC								
	PO	700 [7]					750 [4]		
Block Bradykinin Bronchio- constriction	IV			2 [26]					
	IP		125 [908]						
	IM								
	SC								
	PO								
CNS (Behavioral)	IV						*5 [947]		
	IP	100 [1115]							
	IM								
	SC								
	PO	250 [930]							
Produce Gastric Ulceration	IV								
	IP								
	IM								
	SC		78 [1146]						
	PO								

*Total dose

ALCOHOL, ANHYDROUS

(Ethanol, Ethyl Alcohol)

mg/kg		Mouse	Rat	Guinea Pig	Rabbit	Cat	Dog	Monkey	
Lethal Dose Y–LD$_{50}$ Z–MLD	IV	Y1953 [27]				3945 [33]	5365 [35]		
	IP		Y5000 [29]	Y5560 [4]					
	IM								
	SC	Y8285 [27]					7000		
	PO	Y9488 [27]	Y13,660 [4]		Y9500 [29]		6000		
Increase Brain Serotonin	IV								
	IP		4475 [31]						
	IM								
	SC								
	PO								
Behavioral	IV						3000 [981]		
	IP		15 [32]						
	IM								
	SC								
	PO	3160 [935]					2000 [895]		
CNS	IV		1000 [1208]			4.6 [34]			
	IP								
	IM								
	SC								
	PO								
Paralytic (Anesthetic)	IV								
	IP	4000 [28]		4000 [4]		4000 [4]			
	IM								
	SC								
	PO	8835 [1123]	6000 [1180]	4000 [4]	5000 [4]	4000 [4]			
Hypocalcemic	IV								
	IP								
	IM								
	SC								
	PO		4000 [1207]				2000 [1207]		

ALLOXAN

(Mesoxalylurea, Mesoxalylcarbamide)

mg/kg		Mouse	Rat	Guinea Pig	Rabbit	Cat	Dog	Monkey	
Lethal Dose	IV	Y200 [36]	300 [37]		200 [7]		100 [41]		
Y—LD$_{50}$	IP	Y350 [36]							
Z—MLD	IM								
	SC								
	PO								
Diabetogenic	IV		40 [38]						
	IP		200 [39]						
	IM								
	SC		200 [40]						
	PO					750 [7]			
	IV								
	IP								
	IM								
	SC								
	PO								
	IV								
	IP								
	IM								
	SC								
	PO								
	IV								
	IP								
	IM								
	SC								
	PO								
	IV								
	IP								
	IM								
	SC								
	PO								

mg/kg		Mouse	Rat	Guinea Pig	Rabbit	Cat	Dog	Monkey	
Lethal Dose Y−LD$_{50}$ Z−MLD	IV	Y54 [42]		Y18 [42]	Y18.5				
	IP	Y73 [42]	Y22 [42]						
	IM								
	SC	Y98 [42]	Y23 [42]						
	PO		Y90 [43]						
Analgetic	IV								
	IP								
	IM								
	SC		3 [43]				20		
	PO		10 [43]						
Cardiovascular and Respiratory	IV				1.5 [43]		1.0 [42]		
	IP								
	IM								
	SC								
	PO								
Increase Intestinal Tone	IV						1.0 [43]		
	IP								
	IM								
	SC								
	PO								
	IV								
	IP								
	IM								
	SC								
	PO								
	IV								
	IP								
	IM								
	SC								
	PO								

AMIDEPHRINE

mg/kg		Mouse	Rat	Guinea Pig	Rabbit	Cat	Dog	Monkey	
Lethal Dose Y−LD$_{50}$ Z−MLD	IV	190 [840]							
	IP						4.8 [840]		
	IM								
	SC	Y1990 [840]							
	PO	Y>6000 [840]							
Cardiovascular	IV					4 [840]	0.01 [840]		
	IP	0.3 [840]							
	IM								
	SC								
	PO	5 [840]							
	IV								
	IP								
	IM								
	SC								
	PO								
	IV								
	IP								
	IM								
	SC								
	PO								

IN VITRO

mg %	Cardiac	Vascular	Gut	Uterine	Visceral	Skeletal		

mg/kg		Mouse	Rat	Guinea Pig	Rabbit	Cat	Dog	Monkey	
Lethal Dose Y—LD$_{50}$ Z—MLD	IV	Y184 [49]	Z135 [51]						
	IP		Y248 [52]						
	IM								
	SC	Y350 [49]			417 [56]		300 [57]		
	PO	Y1850 [49]	Y1700	Z925 [4]	Z750 [4]				
Analgetic Antipyretic Anti-inflammatory	IV				50 [50]				
	IP	150 [50]							
	IM								
	SC		200 [50]						
	PO	300 [7]	650 [50]	130 [55]			*265 [24]		
Hypothermic	IV								
	IP				100 [4]				
	IM				100 [4]				
	SC		150 [54]		100 [4]				
	PO		30 [905]						
Decreased Dorsal Root Potential	IV					10 [847]			
	IP								
	IM								
	SC								
	PO								

*Total dose

IN VITRO

mg %	Cardiac	Vascular	Gut	Uterine	Visceral	Skeletal		

AMINOPHYLLINE

(Theophylline ethylenediamine, Carena, Inophylline)

mg/kg		Mouse	Rat	Guinea Pig	Rabbit	Cat	Dog	Monkey	
Lethal Dose Y−LD$_{50}$ Z−MLD	IV		Z190 [77]		Y150 [45]				
	IP								
	IM								
	SC	Z140 [7]							
	PO	Y540							
Cardiovascular	IV		150 [44]		35 [46]	35 [46]	10		
	IP								
	IM								
	SC								
	PO		100 [44]						
Diuretic	IV						20		
	IP								
	IM								
	SC								
	PO		20 [44]						
	IV								
	IP								
	IM								
	SC								
	PO								

IN VITRO

mg %	Cardiac	Vascular	Gut	Uterine	Visceral	Skeletal		
Langendorff (Perfusion)	*5							

*Total mg

α-(l-AMINOPROPYL) PROTOCATECHUYL ALCOHOL

(Ethylnorepinephrine, Butanephrine, Bronkephrine)

mg/kg		Mouse	Rat	Guinea Pig	Rabbit	Cat	Dog	Monkey	
Lethal Dose Y—LD$_{50}$ Z—MLD	IV	Y117 [47]							
	IP								
	IM								
	SC								
	PO								
Bronchiolar Dilatation	IV					1 [48]	1 [47]		
	IP			500 [47]					
	IM								
	SC		80 [47]						
	PO								
Hyperglycemic	IV								
	IP								
	IM								
	SC				10 [47]				
	PO								
	IV								
	IP								
	IM								
	SC								
	PO								

IN VITRO

mg %	Cardiac	Vascular	Gut	Uterine	Visceral	Skeletal		

AMITRIPTYLINE

(Elavil)

mg/kg		Mouse	Rat	Guinea Pig	Rabbit	Cat	Dog	Monkey	
Lethal Dose $Y-LD_{50}$ $Z-MLD$	IV	Y27 [58]			Y9.9 [58]				
	IP	Y76 [58]	Y72 [58]						
	IM								
	SC	Y328 [58]	Y1290 [58]				50 [1210]		
	PO	Y289 [58]	Y530 [58]						
Analeptic to Tetrabenazine	IV								
	IP	1.0 [58]	20 [59]						
	IM								
	SC								
	PO	1.0 [58]							
Adrenolytic Hypothermic	IV						1.2 [58]		
	IP	30 [59]	30 [59]						
	IM								
	SC								
	PO	10 [1071]	10 [1071]						
Behavioral	IV					5 [850]		3 [949]	
	IP	8 [1155]	5.1 [848]						
	IM								
	SC								
	PO							10 [949]	
EEG	IV				2 [835]	0.2 [949]		3 [949]	
	IP								
	IM								
	SC								
	PO								
CNS	IV	6.6 [838]			10 [950]	10 [850]			
	IP								
	IM								
	SC				20 [837]		50 [1210]		
	PO								

AMMONIUM CHLORIDE

(Ammonium Muriate, Sal Ammoniac, Salmiac)

mg/kg		Mouse	Rat	Guinea Pig	Rabbit	Cat	Dog	Monkey	
Lethal Dose Y−LD$_{50}$ Z−MLD	IV			240 [62]					
	IP								
	IM								
	SC	500							
	PO								
Diuretic	IV								
	IP		250 [61]						
	IM								
	SC								
	PO		250						
Medullary Stimulant	IV	150 [4]	150 [4]	150 [4]	150 [4]	150 [4]	150 [4]	150 [4]	
	IP								
	IM								
	SC								
	PO								
	IV								
	IP								
	IM								
	SC								
	PO								

IN VITRO

mg %	Cardiac	Vascular	Gut	Uterine	Visceral	Skeletal		

AMOBARBITAL

(Amytal, Dorminal, Amytalily)

mg/kg		Mouse	Rat	Guinea Pig	Rabbit	Cat	Dog	Monkey	
Lethal Dose Y-LD$_{50}$ Z-MLD	IV	Z135 63	Z90 63	Z80 63	Y75 70	54	61 64		
	IP	200 64	Y115	Z120 63	90 66	Z120 63			
	IM		Z230 4						
	SC	Z280 63	190 68	Z170 63	Z150 63				
	PO		400 63		Y575 71	Y110	125 63		
Anesthetic	IV	54 65	55 63	50 63	40 72	11 24	50	40 63	
	IP	65 66	100 4	60 63	54 66	75	65		
	IM				50	100 4			
	SC	130 63	150	85 63	70 66	100 4	105		
	PO	160 1125	225 69		90 66	100	175 66		
Spinal Cord Depressant	IV					30			
	IP								
	IM								
	SC								
	PO								
Behavioral	IV						1 947		
	IP		5 932						
	IM								
	SC		15 952						
	PO						8 951		
	IV								
	IP								
	IM								
	SC								
	PO								
	IV								
	IP								
	IM								
	SC								
	PO								

AMPHETAMINE

(Benzedrine, Alentol, Ortedrine)

mg/kg		Mouse	Rat	Guinea Pig	Rabbit	Cat	Dog	Monkey	
Lethal Dose Y−LD$_{50}$ Z−MLD	IV	Y25 [73]			25 [52]				
	IP	Y120 [74]	Y125 [80]						
	IM								
	SC	270 [75]	Y160 [81]						
	PO	22 [73]	Y60.5 [82]		Y85		Z20 [83]		
Sympatho-mimetic	IV			0.5	0.5	0.5	0.5		
	IP	90 [936]	10 [7]						
	IM								
	SC		80 [83]						
	PO								
CNS Stimulant	IV				0.75 [87]	1.5	2.5		
	IP								
	IM								
	SC	5 [76]	3 [84]			1.5 [24]	1.69 [942]		
	PO		2						
Antagonize Reserpine Ptosis	IV								
	IP	2.5 [78]							
	IM								
	SC								
	PO	4 [79]							
Increase Spontaneous Motor Activity	IV								
	IP	4 [954]	4 [937]						
	IM								
	SC	1.6 [1101]	0.68 [85]					5 [89]	
	PO		1.25 [936]						
Behavioral	IV					5 [853]	4.3 [1116]		
	IP	2 [874]	2 [834]			7 [1100]			
	IM							*1.15 [90]	
	SC		0.2 [943]				1 [895]		
	PO		3 [934]			2 [953]			

*Total dose

AMPHETAMINE (continued)

mg/kg		Mouse	Rat	Guinea Pig	Rabbit	Cat	Dog	Monkey	
Decrease Tissue Uptake of Norepinephrine	IV					10 [91]			
	IP	10 [910]							
	IM								
	SC								
	PO								
Increase Digestion Time	IV								
	IP		10 [7]						
	IM								
	SC								
	PO								
Hyperthermic Reaction	IV				4 [1182]				
	IP		5 [1136]		15 [820]	15 [820]			
	IM								
	SC		10 [942]						
	PO								
Cardiovascular	IV					0.2 [888]	0.25 [883]		
	IP								
	IM								
	SC								
	PO								

IN VITRO

mg %	Cardiac	Vascular	Gut	Uterine	Visceral	Skeletal		
Antiserotonergic			10 [92]					
Rabbit			2 [1157]					

mg/kg		Mouse	Rat	Guinea Pig	Rabbit	Cat	Dog	Monkey	
Lethal Dose Y−LD$_{50}$ Z−MLD	IV		8 [93]						
	IP								
	IM								
	SC								
	PO								
Cardiovascular	IV		0.0002 [93]			0.0001 [93]	0.0001 [93]		
	IP								
	IM								
	SC					0.0005 [93]			
	PO								
	IV								
	IP								
	IM								
	SC								
	PO								
	IV								
	IP								
	IM								
	SC								
	PO								

IN VITRO

mg %	Cardiac	Vascular	Gut	Uterine	Visceral	Skeletal	Nictitating Membrane	
Contractile	0.0001 [1224]	0.001 [93]	0.001 [93]				0.003 [1236]	

ANILERIDINE

(Leritine, MK89)

mg/kg		Mouse	Rat	Guinea Pig	Rabbit	Cat	Dog	Monkey	
Lethal Dose Y−LD$_{50}$ Z−MLD	IV	*Y25 [58]							
	IP	*Y53 [58]	*Y45 [58]						
	IM								
	SC	*Y100 [58]	*Y163 [58]						
	PO	*Y128 [58]	*Y175 [58]						
Analgetic	IV								
	IP								
	IM							*1.25 [58]	
	SC		*5 [58]				*5 [58]		
	PO		*12 [58]				*5 [58]		
Cardiovascular	IV					2 [94]	2 [94]		
	IP								
	IM								
	SC								
	PO								
Respiratory Depression	IV					4 [94]	4 [94]		
	IP								
	IM								
	SC								
	PO								
	IV								
	IP								
	IM								
	SC								
	PO								
	IV								
	IP								
	IM								
	SC								
	PO								

* as base

mg/kg		Mouse	Rat	Guinea Pig	Rabbit	Cat	Dog	Monkey	
Lethal Dose $Y-LD_{50}$ $Z-MLD$	IV		40 [95]				Y80		
	IP								
	IM								
	SC								
	PO								
Emetic	IV					30 [96]	0.075		
	IP								
	IM								
	SC					30 [96]	0.31 [938]		
	PO						200 [4]		
Morphine Antagonist	IV								
	IP								
	IM								
	SC						1		
	PO								
CNS Stimulant	IV		10 [95]			10-40 [1199]			
	IP								
	IM								
	SC								
	PO								
Bulbocapnine Antagonist	IV	5 [1156]				10 [1156]			
	IP								
	IM								
	SC								
	PO								
	IV								
	IP								
	IM								
	SC								
	PO								

ARTERENOL

(Aktamin, Levophed, Norepinephrine)

mg/kg		Mouse	Rat	Guinea Pig	Rabbit	Cat	Dog	Monkey	
Lethal Dose Y−LD$_{50}$ Z−MLD	IV	Y>2 [896]							
	IP								
	IM								
	SC		Y29 [1128]						
	PO		Y132 [1128]						
Cardiovascular	IV	0.003 [97]	0.003 [97]	0.003 [97]	0.003 [97]	0.003 [97]	0.003 [97]	0.001 [1079]	
	IP								
	IM								
	SC								
	PO								
Behavioral	IV						0.01 [99]		
	IP	4 [939]							
	IM								
	SC	2 [940]							
	PO								
Barbiturate Sleep Potentiation	IV								
	IP	2 [98]							
	IM								
	SC								
	PO								
Antagonize Reserpine Ptosis	IV								
	IP	1 [78]							
	IM								
	SC								
	PO								
Diuretic	IV						0.007 [866]		
	IP								
	IM								
	SC		0.25 [151]		1.0 [863]				
	PO								

mg/kg		Mouse	Rat	Guinea Pig	Rabbit	Cat	Dog	Monkey	
Bronchiolar Dilatation	IV								
	IP								
	IM								
	SC			0.4 [1081]					
	PO								
Metabolic	IV								
	IP								
	IM								
	SC		1 [864]		1 [863]				
	PO								
	IV								
	IP								
	IM								
	SC								
	PO								
	IV								
	IP								
	IM								
	SC								
	PO								

IN VITRO

mg %	Cardiac	Vascular	Gut	Uterine	Visceral	Skeletal	Trachea	
Langendorff	*0.1							
Guinea Pig							0.006 [1157]	
Rabbit	0.12 [1157]	0.0003 [1157]	0.02 [1157]					
Rat				0.003 [1157]				

*Total mg

ATROPINE
(Atropisol)

mg/kg		Mouse	Rat	Guinea Pig	Rabbit	Cat	Dog	Monkey	
Lethal Dose $Y-LD_{50}$ $Z-MLD$	IV	Y90 [100]			71 [107]	Z30 [109]	100 [104]		
	IP	Y250 [101]	Y280 [101]	Y400 [101]			175 [104]		
	IM								
	SC	Y900 [101]	750 [101]	450 [104]	375 [107]	140 [104]	225 [104]		
	PO	Y400 [102]	Y750 [101]	Y1100 [101]	1450 [107]				
Anticholinergic	IV	1 [1197]			2	2 [109]	1		
	IP	0.33 [915]	0.5 [103]						
	IM			5	0.11 [101]				
	SC	0.05 [101]	3 [101]			0.6 [110]	0.5		
	PO	0.55 [101]	10 [101]						
Preanesthetic Medication	IV								
	IP								
	IM					1.0 [557]	2.75 [557]		
	SC	0.05 [97]	0.05 [97]	0.05 [97]	0.05 [97]	0.05 [557]	0.1	0.05 [97]	
	PO			1 [105]					
CNS (EEG)	IV				3 [108]	4 [112]			
	IP		6 [1158]			4 [112]			
	IM							1.5 [945]	
	SC		5 [1159]				7.2 [1160]		
	PO								
Behavioral	IV				0.5 [1161]		1 [915]	0.3 [1163]	
	IP	10 [1116]	15 [106]			3.5 [1100]			
	IM					1.5 [945]		1.5 [945]	
	SC	10 [856]	5 [941]			10 [944]	0.5 [1162]		
	PO	20 [935]				50 [945]			
Antiserotonergic	IV			10 [92]					
	IP								
	IM								
	SC								
	PO								

mg/kg		Mouse	Rat	Guinea Pig	Rabbit	Cat	Dog	Monkey	
Protect Against Coronary Occlusion	IV						0.1 [7]		
	IP								
	IM								
	SC								
	PO								
Block Superior Cervical Ganglion Transmission	IV					2.5 [113]			
	IP								
	IM								
	SC								
	PO								
Anticonvulsant	IV								
	IP								
	IM								
	SC	3 [957]							
	PO								
Decrease Dopamine Uptake (Brain)	IV								
	IP						50 [1240]		
	IM								
	SC								
	PO								

IN VITRO

mg %	Cardiac	Vascular	Gut	Uterine	Visceral	Skeletal		
Anticholinergic	0.1		0.01 [101]	0.1	0.01			
Antiserotonergic Rat			1.0 [92]					
Antiserotonergic G.P.			0.5 [92]					
Langendorff	*0.05 [1157]							

*Total mg.

ATROPINE METHYLNITRATE

(Eumydrin, Harvatrate, Metropine)

mg/kg		Mouse	Rat	Guinea Pig	Rabbit	Cat	Dog	Monkey	
Lethal Dose	IV								
Y—LD$_{50}$	IP	Y 250							
Z—MLD	IM								
	SC								
	PO								
Cardiovascular	IV			2		1.5	3		
	IP								
	IM								
	SC								
	PO								
CNS	IV					10 114			
	IP								
	IM								
	SC								
	PO								
	IV								
	IP								
	IM								
	SC								
	PO								

IN VITRO

mg %	Cardiac	Vascular	Gut	Uterine	Visceral	Skeletal		
Anticholinergic	10		10					

AZACYCLONOL

(Frenquel, MER-17, Gamma-Pipradrol)

mg/kg		Mouse	Rat	Guinea Pig	Rabbit	Cat	Dog	Monkey	
Lethal Dose $Y-LD_{50}$ $Z-MLD$	IV	Y177 [115]					45 [117]		
	IP	Y220 [115]							
	IM								
	SC	Y350 [115]							
	PO	Y650 [115]							
Decreased Spontaneous Motor Activity	IV	93 [116]							
	IP								
	IM								
	SC	213 [116]							
	PO	520 [116]							
Hexobarbital Sleep Potentiation	IV								
	IP	78 [117]							
	IM								
	SC	71 [116]							
	PO	100 [118]							
Cardiovascular	IV						32 [117]		
	IP								
	IM								
	SC								
	PO	300 [119]							
Hypothermic	IV								
	IP								
	IM				10 [120]				
	SC								
	PO								
	IV								
	IP								
	IM								
	SC								
	PO								

BARBITAL

(Veronal, Medinal, Barbitone)

mg/kg		Mouse	Rat	Guinea Pig	Rabbit	Cat	Dog	Monkey	
Lethal Dose $Y-LD_{50}$ $Z-MLD$	IV	440 [27]			350 [66]				
	IP	Y760 [122]	300 [66]		375 [128]				
	IM								
	SC	340 [66]	330 [66]		350 [66]	300			
	PO	600	400		Z275 [129]	275 [66]	350 [66]		
Anesthetic	IV	234 [65]			175	200	220		
	IP	300 [124]	190 [125]				250		
	IM								
	SC		200 [126]		110 [66]				
	PO		190 [125]		110 [66]	150 [66]			
Hypnotic	IV	275 [956]			130				
	IP		145 [127]						
	IM								
	SC	25 [958]							
	PO					*200 [24]	*550 [24]		
Behavioral	IV						125	0.6-10 [1178]	
	IP	70 [1131]	240 [1095]						
	IM								
	SC								
	PO	100 [935]					2000 [30]		
Anticonvulsant	IV								
	IP	15.2 [955]							
	IM								
	SC	100 [957]							
	PO		30 [959]						
	IV								
	IP								
	IM								
	SC								
	PO								

*Total dose

mg/kg		Mouse	Rat	Guinea Pig	Rabbit	Cat	Dog	Monkey	
Lethal Dose Y−LD$_{50}$ Z−MLD	IV		Z 20 [53]		17 [86]	50 [86]	26 [86]		
	IP	Y500							
	IM								
	SC		Y 178 [82]	55 [86]	55 [82]	38 [82]	15 [86]		
	PO		335 [82]		170 [82]		90		
Cardiovascular	IV			10			7.5		
	IP								
	IM								
	SC		35 [82]						
	PO								
	IV								
	IP								
	IM								
	SC								
	PO								
	IV								
	IP								
	IM								
	SC								
	PO								

IN VITRO

mg %	Cardiac	Vascular	Gut	Uterine	Visceral	Skeletal		
Spasmogenic	5	2	3 [88]		10			
Guinea Pig			4 [1157]					

BEMEGRIDE

(Megimide, Mikedimide, Eukraton)

mg/kg		Mouse	Rat	Guinea Pig	Rabbit	Cat	Dog	Monkey	
Lethal Dose Y–LD$_{50}$ Z–MLD	IV	Y20 [111]	Y16.3 [121]	Y26.5 [131]	Y25 [121]				
	IP	Y45 [111]	Y23.5 [121]						
	IM								
	SC	Y43 [121]	Y30.5 [962]						
	PO	Y100 [111]							
Analeptic	IV	10 [111]		10 [131]	1.0 [132]	14 [97]	10 [133]		
	IP	10 [961]	30 [123]	15 [961]		14 [97]	20 [97]		
	IM								
	SC	25 [964]							
	PO								
Convulsant	IV	20.1 [121]	9.5 [121]	18.5 [131]	5.5 [121]	4.5 [134]			
	IP	20 [961]	20 [130]	17.5 [961]					
	IM								
	SC	43 [121]							
	PO								
CNS (EEG)	IV	10 [963]			3 [963]	2 [854]			
	IP								
	IM								
	SC								
	PO	25 [960]							
Decrease Presynaptic Inhibition	IV				10 [1103]				
	IP								
	IM								
	SC								
	PO								
	IV								
	IP								
	IM								
	SC								
	PO								

BENACTYZINE

(Suavitil, Parasan, Cafron)

mg/kg		Mouse	Rat	Guinea Pig	Rabbit	Cat	Dog	Monkey	
Lethal Dose Y−LD$_{50}$ Z−MLD	IV				15 135				
	IP	115 135	115 135	115 135	115 135				
	IM								
	SC	Y250 136							
	PO	Y350 119							
Behavioral	IV				1 132	4.7 145	1.8 915		
	IP	22 137	50 106						
	IM				0.1 967				
	SC	50 138	20 143		1.5 941	6 135			
	PO								
Barbiturate Sleep Potentiation	IV				5 141				
	IP	5 141							
	IM								
	SC	5 142		30 142	25 142				
	PO			50 142					
Anticonvulsant	IV				1 132				
	IP	10 139		15 132					
	IM	2 140							
	SC								
	PO								
Anticholinergic	IV				0.5 135	0.1 135			
	IP	6 915	24 144						
	IM								
	SC	2 839							
	PO								
EEG	IV				0.5 969	2 968			
	IP								
	IM								
	SC								
	PO								

BENZATROPINE

(Cogentin, Amilyt, Cobretin)

mg/kg		Mouse	Rat	Guinea Pig	Rabbit	Cat	Dog	Monkey	
Lethal Dose $Y-LD_{50}$ $Z-MLD$	IV	Y25 58							
	IP								
	IM								
	SC	Y103 58	Y353 58						
	PO	Y94 58							
Anticholinergic	IV				0.2 839	1 58			
	IP								
	IM								
	SC	0.95 839	1.9 839						
	PO								
Antagonize Tremorine	IV								
	IP	1.5 58							
	IM								
	SC								
	PO								
Increased EEG Arousal Threshold	IV				0.2 831				
	IP								
	IM								
	SC								
	PO								

IN VITRO

mg %	Cardiac	Vascular	Gut	Uterine	Visceral	Skeletal		

BISHYDROXYCOUMARIN

(Dicumarol, Dicoumarin, Melitoxin)

mg/kg		Mouse	Rat	Guinea Pig	Rabbit	Cat	Dog	Monkey	
Lethal Dose	IV	Y64 [146]	Y52 [146]	Y59 [146]			40		
Y−LD$_{50}$	IP	Y350							
Z−MLD	IM								
	SC								
	PO	Y233 [146]	Y542 [146]						
Anticoagulant	IV						10 [7]		
	IP								
	IM								
	SC								
	PO		8 [147]				20		
	IV								
	IP								
	IM								
	SC								
	PO								
	IV								
	IP								
	IM								
	SC								
	PO								

IN VITRO

mg %	Cardiac	Vascular	Gut	Uterine	Visceral	Skeletal		

BRADYKININ

mg/kg		Mouse	Rat	Guinea Pig	Rabbit	Cat	Dog	Monkey	
Lethal Dose Y−LD$_{50}$ Z−MLD	IV								
	IP								
	IM								
	SC								
	PO								
	IV								
	IP								
	IM								
	SC								
	PO								
	IV								
	IP								
	IM								
	SC								
	PO								
	IV								
	IP								
	IM								
	SC								
	PO								

IN VITRO

mg %	Cardiac	Vascular	Gut	Uterine	Visceral	Skeletal		
Guinea Pig			0.002 [1157]					
Rat		0.9 [1204]						

mg/kg		Mouse	Rat	Guinea Pig	Rabbit	Cat	Dog	Monkey	
Lethal Dose Y−LD$_{50}$ Z−MLD	IV	Y20 [148]							
	IP	Y49 [149]							
	IM								
	SC	Y72 [148]							
	PO	Y400 [148]						>400 [149]	
Sympatholytic	IV	12.5 [148]	5 [150]		10 [1133]	15 [153]	5 [154]		
	IP								
	IM								
	SC								
	PO		400 [148]					200 [148]	
Neuromuscular Block	IV								
	IP								
	IM								
	SC					100 [148]		50 [148]	
	PO								
Increased Norepinephrine in Liver, Heart and Kidney	IV								
	IP			50 [152]					
	IM								
	SC								
	PO								
Diuretic	IV								
	IP								
	IM								
	SC		100 [151]						
	PO								
Prevent Guanethidine Depletion of Heart Catechol Amines	IV		5 [150]						
	IP								
	IM								
	SC								
	PO								

mg/kg		Mouse	Rat	Guinea Pig	Rabbit	Cat	Dog	Monkey	
Bronchiolar Dilatation	IV								
	IP								
	IM								
	SC			20 [1081]					
	PO								
Cardiovascular Reflex	IV						10 [1177]		
	IP		10 [1243]						
	IM								
	SC								
	PO								
	IV								
	IP								
	IM								
	SC								
	PO								
	IV								
	IP								
	IM								
	SC								
	PO								

IN VITRO

mg %	Cardiac	Vascular	Gut	Uterine	Visceral	Skeletal		
Finkleman [812]			0.3 [148]					
Rabbit Ear		0.1 [148]						
Guinea Pig	0.5		20 [148]	15 [148]				
Rat Diaphragm						40 [148]		

BUFOTENINE

(Mappine, N-N-dimethylserotonin)

mg/kg		Mouse	Rat	Guinea Pig	Rabbit	Cat	Dog	Monkey	
Lethal Dose Y—LD_{50} Z—MLD	IV								
	IP		125 [155]						
	IM								
	SC								
	PO								
Behavioral	IV				1 [157]		1 [160]	10 [161]	
	IP	5 [156]	5 [156]						
	IM							10 [161]	
	SC		5 [156]						
	PO								
Cardiovascular	IV				0.1 [158]	0.1 [158]	0.05 [158]		
	IP		0.1 [155]						
	IM								
	SC								
	PO								
EEG (synchronization)	IV				0.08 [159]	5 [842]			
	IP								
	IM								
	SC				2.5 [156]				
	PO								
	IV								
	IP								
	IM								
	SC								
	PO								
	IV								
	IP								
	IM								
	SC								
	PO								

BULBOCAPNINE

mg/kg		Mouse	Rat	Guinea Pig	Rabbit	Cat	Dog	Monkey	
Lethal Dose Y–LD$_{50}$ Z–MLD	IV								
	IP								
	IM								
	SC	Y195 [162]							
	PO								
Catatonic	IV						40 [169]		
	IP	125 [163]	50 [165]			20 [1156]		10 [170]	
	IM								
	SC	70 [164]			100 [970]	40 [971]			
	PO								
Cardiovascular	IV					8 [167]			
	IP								
	IM								
	SC		75 [166]						
	PO								
Antagonize 5-HT and Catechol Amines	IV				90 [167]	30 [168]	60 [167]		
	IP								
	IM								
	SC								
	PO								
Convulsant	IV								
	IP								
	IM							40 [161]	
	SC								
	PO								
EEG	IV					25 [842]			
	IP								
	IM								
	SC								
	PO								

(N-Benzyl-N'N''-dimethylguanidine)

mg/kg		Mouse	Rat	Guinea Pig	Rabbit	Cat	Dog	Monkey	
Lethal Dose $Y-LD_{50}$ $Z-MLD$	IV	Y12 [171]							
	IP	Y150 [171]							
	IM								
	SC	Y260 [171]							
	PO	Y520 [171]							
Sympatholytic	IV				0.5 [171]	0.3 [171]	0.65 [171]	10 [171]	
	IP								
	IM								
	SC					2.5 [171]			
	PO					2.5 [171]	5 [171]		
Neuromuscular Block	IV					15 [171]	15 [171]	15 [171]	
	IP								
	IM								
	SC					100 [171]			
	PO								
	IV								
	IP								
	IM								
	SC								
	PO								

IN VITRO

mg %	Cardiac	Vascular	Gut	Uterine	Visceral	Skeletal		
Adrenolytic		*0.065 [171]						
Sympathomimetic		*0.3 [171]			1 [171]			

*Total mg

CAFFEINE

(Coffeine, Guaranine, Methyltheobromine)

mg/kg		Mouse	Rat	Guinea Pig	Rabbit	Cat	Dog	Monkey	
Lethal Dose Y–LD$_{50}$ Z–MLD	IV	Y100 172	Y105 172		90 109	Z90 109	Y175 183		
	IP	250	Y245 109	Z235 109		Z190 109			
	IM				200 182				
	SC	185 195	Y250 178	Z220 109	275 182	150 109	110 182		
	PO	†Y1200 960	Y200		355 182	Z125 109	Z145 109		
CNS (Stimulant)	IV				25	40 854			
	IP	7.5 174	50 179						
	IM	20 175				*125 24	125 24		
	SC	20 176	15 180			*125 24	50 24		
	PO	100 960							
Antiseroton-ergic	IV			30 92					
	IP	20 177	40 181						
	IM								
	SC		40 181						
	PO								
Behavioral	IV								
	IP	16 1131	150 972					200 185	
	IM								
	SC	20 940							
	PO	200 935	100 973			25 953			
Analeptic	IV				40		50		
	IP								
	IM								
	SC	200 964							
	PO								
EEG	IV				*450 974	10 184			
	IP								
	IM								
	SC								
	PO								

*Total dose

†Housed individually

mg/kg		Mouse	Rat	Guinea Pig	Rabbit	Cat	Dog	Monkey	
Decurariza-tion	IV					*210　　7			
	IP								
	IM								
	SC								
	PO								
	IV								
	IP								
	IM								
	SC								
	PO								
	IV								
	IP								
	IM								
	SC								
	PO								
	IV								
	IP								
	IM								
	SC								
	PO								

*Total dose

IN VITRO

mg %	Cardiac	Vascular	Gut	Uterine	Visceral	Skeletal		
Antiserotonergic			10　　92					
Langendorff	*1　　1157							

*Total mg.

CALCIUM CHLORIDE

mg/kg		Mouse	Rat	Guinea Pig	Rabbit	Cat	Dog	Monkey	
Lethal Dose $Y-LD_{50}$ $Z-MLD$	IV		Z169 [186]		274 [109]	249 [109]	274 [109]		
	IP		Y500 [187]						
	IM								
	SC				472 [109]	249 [109]	274 [109]		
	PO		Y4000 [187]		1384 [109]				
Convulsant	IV								
	IP								
	IM								
	SC		1000 [188]						
	PO								
Magnesium Sulfate Antagonist	IV				150				
	IP								
	IM								
	SC								
	PO								
	IV								
	IP								
	IM								
	SC								
	PO								

IN VITRO

mg %	Cardiac	Vascular	Gut	Uterine	Visceral	Skeletal		

mg/kg		Mouse	Rat	Guinea Pig	Rabbit	Cat	Dog	Monkey	
Lethal Dose Y−LD$_{50}$ Z−MLD	IV	Y0.3 [13]	Y0.1 [13]	0.045 [189]					
	IP								
	IM								
	SC	Y3 [13]	Y4 [13]	0.08 [190]					
	PO	Y15 [13]	Y40 [13]						
Cholinergic	IV				0.002 [14]	0.03	0.03		
	IP								
	IM								
	SC				0.1 [14]		0.01 [14]		
	PO				2 [14]		0.25 [14]		
Nicotinic (Atropinized Animal)	IV					0.1	0.1		
	IP								
	IM								
	SC								
	PO								
	IV								
	IP								
	IM								
	SC								
	PO								

IN VITRO

mg %	Cardiac	Vascular	Gut	Uterine	Visceral	Skeletal		
Guinea Pig	0.008 [1157]		0.04 [1157]					
Rat				0.02 [1157]				
Langendorff	*0.1 [1157]							

*Total mg.

CARISOPRODOL

(Soma, Somadril, Carisoma)

mg/kg		Mouse	Rat	Guinea Pig	Rabbit	Cat	Dog	Monkey	
Lethal Dose Y−LD$_{50}$ Z−MLD	IV	165 [191]	Y450 [115]		Y124 [845]				
	IP								
	IM								
	SC								
	PO		Y1320 [115]						
Analgetic	IV	10 [191]			10 [191]				
	IP								
	IM								
	SC								
	PO		130 [117]	100 [192]					
Block EEG Desynchronization from Afferent Nerve Stimulation	IV				10	10 [193]			
	IP								
	IM								
	SC								
	PO								
Spinal Cord Depressant	IV					10 [841]	30 [191]		
	IP								
	IM								
	SC	100 [142]							
	PO	225 [1146]	305 [975]						
Barbiturate Sleep Potentiation	IV								
	IP								
	IM								
	SC					100 [142]			
	PO			100 [142]					
Paralytic	IV				15.7 [845]	5 [845]			
	IP								
	IM								
	SC								
	PO								

mg/kg		Mouse	Rat	Guinea Pig	Rabbit	Cat	Dog	Monkey	
Lethal Dose Y−LD$_{50}$ Z−MLD	IV								
	IP	Z650 [194]	500						
	IM								
	SC	825 [195]	Y620 [196]		1000 [198]				
	PO		Y500 [197]		1400 [199]	Z440 [201]	1100 [203]		
Anesthetic	IV					300 [1232]	125		
	IP	400	300 [197]	400 [1164]					
	IM								
	SC						150		
	PO					250	500		
Cardiovascular and Respiratory	IV					25.8 [34]	125		
	IP								
	IM								
	SC								
	PO								
Behavioral and EEG	IV				30 [200]	30 [202]	40 [951]		
	IP	64 [1155]							
	IM								
	SC								
	PO	200 [935]			30 [200]				
Increased Serotonin (Brain)	IV								
	IP		300 [31]						
	IM								
	SC								
	PO								
	IV								
	IP								
	IM								
	SC								
	PO								

69

α-CHLORALOSE

(Glucochloral, Chloralosane, Somio)

mg/kg		Mouse	Rat	Guinea Pig	Rabbit	Cat	Dog	Monkey	
Lethal Dose Y−LD$_{50}$ Z−MLD	IV						120 [207]		
	IP	Y200 [204]				150 [207]			
	IM								
	SC		200		80 [206]				
	PO		400			600 [207]	600 [207]		
Anesthetic	IV				120	75 [208]	100 [209]		
	IP	114 [204]	55 [205]			50			
	IM								
	SC								
	PO								
Increased Serotonin (Brain)	IV								
	IP		100 [31]						
	IM								
	SC								
	PO								
	IV								
	IP								
	IM								
	SC								
	PO								

IN VITRO

mg %	Cardiac	Vascular	Gut	Uterine	Visceral	Skeletal		

mg/kg		Mouse	Rat	Guinea Pig	Rabbit	Cat	Dog	Monkey	
Lethal Dose $Y-LD_{50}$ $Z-MLD$	IV	Y95 [210]	Y165 [115]		Y36 [845]				
	IP	Y268 [210]							
	IM								
	SC	Y530 [210]	Y800 [210]						
	PO	Y720 [210]	Y2000 [115]		Y590 [1123]		Y1000		
Sedative	IV	30 [211]					*10 [212]		
	IP	50 [211]							
	IM							100 [976]	
	SC	94 [211]			25 [978]				
	PO	224 [211]	49 [211]			6 [557]	7.5 [557]	1 [213]	
Hypnotic	IV	72 [211]					80 [964]		
	IP	210 [211]							
	IM								
	SC	530 [211]							
	PO	740 [211]		50 [978]			80 [213]		
Anticonvulsant	IV	6.2 [881]				1 [1117]		18	
	IP	40 [1115]							
	IM								
	SC	29 [920]							
	PO	100 [211]	12 [1072]						
Ataxic	IV				17.5 [845]	10 [845]			
	IP	40 [1115]							
	IM							100 [976]	
	SC								
	PO	152 [881]	6.6 [1125]			10 [1165]	10 [211]	20 [211]	
Behavioral	IV								
	IP	8 [1155]	15 [829]			10 [1147]			
	IM							20 [976]	
	SC								
	PO	50 [935]	60 [977]			10 [1108]		1 [1123]	

*Total dose

CHLORISONDAMINE

(Ecolid, SU-3088)

mg/kg		Mouse	Rat	Guinea Pig	Rabbit	Cat	Dog	Monkey	
Lethal Dose Y−LD$_{50}$ Z−MLD	IV	Y24 [214]	Y28 [215]						
	IP								
	IM								
	SC								
	PO	Y401 [214]							
Ganglionic Block	IV					0.32 [215]	0.5		
	IP								
	IM		5 [867]						
	SC								
	PO						20 [215]		
Cardiovascular	IV		1.0 [216]		0.32 [216]		0.3 [215]	1.0 [216]	
	IP								
	IM								
	SC		0.11 [916]						
	PO								
Metabolic	IV								
	IP								
	IM								
	SC		5 [884]						
	PO								

IN VITRO

mg %	Cardiac	Vascular	Gut	Uterine	Visceral	Skeletal		
Anticholinergic			1.0 [215]					

N-(2-CHLOROETHYL) DIBENZYLAMINE

(Dibenamine)

mg/kg		Mouse	Rat	Guinea Pig	Rabbit	Cat	Dog	Monkey	
Lethal Dose $Y-LD_{50}$ $Z-MLD$	IV								
	IP								
	IM								
	SC	Y800 [217]							
	PO								
Adrenolytic	IV		20 [218]		50 [220]	30 [220]	15 [220]		
	IP		10 [219]						
	IM								
	SC								
	PO								
Inhibit Analeptic Effect of Amphetamine	IV				15				
	IP								
	IM								
	SC								
	PO								
Cardiovascular	IV					20 [821]	10 [1177]		
	IP								
	IM								
	SC								
	PO								

IN VITRO

mg %	Cardiac	Vascular	Gut	Uterine	Visceral	Skeletal		
Antiserotonergic			0.03 [92]					

CHLORPHENIRAMINE

(Chlor-Trimeton, Allergisan, Piriton)

mg/kg		Mouse	Rat	Guinea Pig	Rabbit	Cat	Dog	Monkey	
Lethal Dose Y—LD$_{50}$ Z—MLD	IV	39.6 [221]					98 [221]		
	IP	76.7 [221]							
	IM								
	SC	104.0 [221]		101.1 [221]					
	PO	142 [221]		186 [222]					
Antihistaminic	IV			1.16 [221]		0.1 [97]	5		
	IP								
	IM					0.1 [97]	0.1 [97]		
	SC			5			5		
	PO			0.13 [222]		0.1 [97]	0.1 [97]		
CNS (Stimulant)	IV								
	IP								
	IM								
	SC								
	PO	12 [222]				12 [222]			
Behavioral	IV								
	IP	25 [1131]	23 [848]						
	IM								
	SC								
	PO								

IN VITRO

mg %	Cardiac	Vascular	Gut	Uterine	Visceral	Skeletal		
Antihistaminic			0.0001 [223]					

CHLORPROMAZINE
(Largactil, Thorazine, Megaphen)

mg/kg		Mouse	Rat	Guinea Pig	Rabbit	Cat	Dog	Monkey	
Lethal Dose $Y-LD_{50}$ $Z-MLD$	IV	Y26 557	Y29 115		Y16 235		Y30 228		
	IP	Y92 82	Y74 228						
	IM								
	SC	Y300 983	Y542 82						
	PO	Y319 82	Y493 82						
Sedative	IV				10 236	2.5 97	2.5 97	0.3 248	
	IP	12.5 892	8 59					5 161	
	IM					5 557	4 557	0.3 248	
	SC	25	20 88	50 978		1.5 1232	4	0.63 249	
	PO	96 1122		25 978		3.3 97	3.3 97	4.74 250	
Behavioral	IV				7 60	3 823	0.2 243		
	IP	6 224	4 229			2 926		5 185	
	IM	3 175	1 230			5 980	5 244		
	SC	10 225	5 231	20 978	5 979		1 245	0.3 977	
	PO	15.7 226	7 232	100 1166		6 1108	20 246	10 977	
EEG	IV				3 237	2 239	1 247	1 247	
	IP		5 1069	5 234	0.5 238	15 240			
	IM								
	SC				5 156				
	PO					10 1165			
Cardiovascular	IV		2.5 218		10 236	4 241	5 88		
	IP								
	IM					0.5 242			
	SC		2 986						
	PO								
Barbiturate Sleep Potentiation	IV	1	10 233						
	IP	4.1 227							
	IM								
	SC	50 142			25 142	2.2 1232			
	PO	8 983		100 105					

CHLORPROMAZINE (continued)

mg/kg		Mouse	Rat	Guinea Pig	Rabbit	Cat	Dog	Monkey	
Anticonvulsant	IV								
	IP	20 [251]	10 [982]	10 [982]					
	IM								
	SC	60 [252]		50 [978]	5 [88]	2 [110]			
	PO	100 [142]							
Adrenolytic	IV		0.026 [253]				0.5		
	IP								
	IM						0.5		
	SC					50 [88]			
	PO						10		
Analgetic	IV				2 [844]				
	IP	5 [1119]							
	IM	0.79 [908]							
	SC			50 [978]					
	PO	5 [844]							
Hypothermic	IV								
	IP	10 [985]	2 [1104]	5 [984]					
	IM		5 [1241]						
	SC	5 [983]	25 [986]						
	PO	12 [983]							

IN VITRO

mg %	Cardiac	Vascular	Gut	Uterine	Visceral	Skeletal		
Langendorff	1.0 [88]							
Antiserotonergic			0.01 [92]					
Rabbit Atria	100 [88]							

mg/kg		Mouse	Rat	Guinea Pig	Rabbit	Cat	Dog	Monkey	
Lethal Dose Y−LD$_{50}$ Z−MLD	IV	Y1120 [58]					Y1000 [58]		
	IP	1400 [255]	Y1386 [58]						
	IM								
	SC								
	PO	Y8510 [58]	Y10000 [58]						
Diuretic	IV						6 [58]		
	IP		100 [58]						
	IM								
	SC								
	PO		100 [58]				3 [58]		
Cardiovascular	IV						25 [1217]		
	IP								
	IM								
	SC								
	PO								
	IV								
	IP								
	IM								
	SC								
	PO								

IN VITRO

mg %	Cardiac	Vascular	Gut	Uterine	Visceral	Skeletal		

COCAINE

mg/kg		Mouse	Rat	Guinea Pig	Rabbit	Cat	Dog	Monkey	
Lethal Dose $Y-LD_{50}$ $Z-MLD$	IV	Z 30 [256]	Y 17.5 [258]	Z 20 [67]	Y 17 [259]	Z 14.6 [63]			
	IP	Y 150	Y 70 [259]	Z 60 [67]					
	IM								
	SC	100 [257]	Y 250 [259]	Z 50 [67]	Z 126	Z 31.9 [63]	Z 35 [63]		
	PO								
Cardiovascular	IV			1	1 [261]	5	2 [261]		
	IP		20						
	IM						10 [263]		
	SC				1.5 [7]	20	20		
	PO								
CNS Stimulant	IV				1.3 [262]	1.3 [262]			
	IP	55 [251]							
	IM	10 [175]							
	SC	20 [176]		10 [978]	10 [978]				
	PO								
Convulsant	IV		10.5 [260]						
	IP					50 [948]			
	IM								
	SC				80				
	PO								
Counteract Bulbocapnine Catatonia	IV								
	IP								
	IM								
	SC							5 [170]	
	PO								
Decreased Norepinephrine in Heart, Spleen, and Adrenals	IV					5 [91]			
	IP								
	IM								
	SC								
	PO								

mg/kg		Mouse	Rat	Guinea Pig	Rabbit	Cat	Dog	Monkey	
Reserpine Antagonist	IV				6.8 988				
	IP	40 264							
	IM								
	SC								
	PO								
Hyperthermic	IV								
	IP								
	IM				25				
	SC								
	PO								
Behavioral	IV								
	IP	25 987							
	IM								
	SC	16 1101	10 988						
	PO								
Diuretic	IV								
	IP								
	IM								
	SC							10 854	
	PO								

IN VITRO

mg %	Cardiac	Vascular	Gut	Uterine	Visceral	Skeletal		
Potentiate Epinephrine	0.05 265	0.01	0.14 1157		1			
Block Dopamine	*0.008 266							
Antiserotonergic			10 92					

*Total mg

CODEINE

(Methylmorphine)

mg/kg		Mouse	Rat	Guinea Pig	Rabbit	Cat	Dog	Monkey	
Lethal Dose $Y-LD_{50}$ $Z-MLD$	IV	Y68 267	Y55 267		Y60 990				
	IP	Y130 17	Y102 268						
	IM								
	SC	Y183 267	Y332 267		Y32 270		150 989		
	PO	Y395 267	Y542 267	Z120 109	100 109		200 109		
Analgetic	IV	25.5 267	6.2 267		10 191				
	IP	40	63						
	IM		14.8 267						
	SC	5.6 908	17 908	28 991			5		
	PO	97 267	22.5 267		10 271		31 1114		
Antitussive	IV		10 269			2.3 989			
	IP			2 948					
	IM								
	SC		50 269				2.2 24		
	PO			42 1124			2.2 24		
Behavioral	IV	10 191							
	IP	100 989				50 948			
	IM								
	SC								
	PO								
Emetic	IV								
	IP								
	IM								
	SC						6.5 267		
	PO						5.0 267		
Depress Spinal Reflexes	IV					12 990	5 894		
	IP								
	IM								
	SC								
	PO						20 894		

mg/kg		Mouse	Rat	Guinea Pig	Rabbit	Cat	Dog	Monkey	
Lethal Dose $Y-LD_{50}$ $Z-MLD$	IV		Y1.7 275		Z5.5 277	Y0.25 279			
	IP	Y3.5 272	4 275						
	IM								
	SC	Y3.1 273	Y4 276		Z7.5 277	0.8 109	0.57 109		
	PO	66.6 272				0.13 109	0.13 109		
Cardiovascular	IV					5 275			
	IP								
	IM								
	SC				15 278				
	PO								
Arrest Mitotic Division	IV								
	IP								
	IM								
	SC	2 274							
	PO								
	IV								
	IP								
	IM								
	SC								
	PO								

IN VITRO

mg %	Cardiac	Vascular	Gut	Uterine	Visceral	Skeletal		

CYPROHEPTADINE

(Periactin)

mg/kg		Mouse	Rat	Guinea Pig	Rabbit	Cat	Dog	Monkey	
Lethal Dose	IV	Y23 [58]			4 [58]				
Y—LD$_{50}$	IP	Y55 [58]	Y52 [58]						
Z—MLD	IM								
	SC	Y107 [58]							
	PO	Y125 [58]	Y295 [58]				50 [58]		
Antiserotonin	IV						0.1 [58]		
	IP								
	IM								
	SC		0.05 [58]						
	PO		0.08 [58]						
Antihistaminic	IV						0.05 [82]		
	IP			0.25 [58]					
	IM								
	SC								
	PO								
	IV								
	IP								
	IM								
	SC								
	PO								

IN VITRO

mg %	Cardiac	Vascular	Gut	Uterine	Visceral	Skeletal		
Antiserotonergic					4×10^{-5} [58]			
Rat			0.017 [1157]					

DECAMETHONIUM

(Syncurine, C-10, Curam)

mg/kg		Mouse	Rat	Guinea Pig	Rabbit	Cat	Dog	Monkey	
Lethal Dose $Y-LD_{50}$ $Z-MLD$	IV	Y0.75 [280]			Y0.2 [281]				
	IP								
	IM								
	SC								
	PO								
Neuromuscular Block	IV	0.17 [280]			0.1 [281]	0.015	0.2 [282]	0.1 [283]	
	IP								
	IM								
	SC								
	PO								
Behavioral	IV								
	IP		0.8 [61]						
	IM								
	SC								
	PO								
	IV								
	IP								
	IM								
	SC								
	PO								

IN VITRO

mg %	Cardiac	Vascular	Gut	Uterine	Visceral	Skeletal		
Rat						1.5 [1157]		

DEXAMPHETAMINE

(Dexedrine, Amsustain, Dephadren)

mg/kg		Mouse	Rat	Guinea Pig	Rabbit	Cat	Dog	Monkey	
Lethal Dose $Y-LD_{50}$ $Z-MLD$	IV	Y14.3							
	IP	Y72.2 [284]							
	IM								
	SC	Y84 [285]	Y200						
	PO	Y37 [82]	Y80 [82]				Z6.4 [82]	Z32 [82]	
Cardiovascular	IV	0.4	0.4	0.4	0.4	0.35	0.4		
	IP								
	IM								
	SC								
	PO								
CNS Stimulant	IV				0.5 [108]	1.0 [184]	2.5		
	IP	10 [286]				3 [993]			
	IM								
	SC		3 [180]				2.5		
	PO		1 [232]						
Behavioral	IV				5 [288]		1 [945]		
	IP	2 [992]	2 [287]					0.2 [185]	
	IM							0.5 [289]	
	SC	5 [933]							
	PO	20 [935]	1 [232]						
Antagonize Adrenolytic Action of Bretylium	IV					0.35 [153]			
	IP								
	IM								
	SC								
	PO								
Analeptic	IV				10		20		
	IP								
	IM								
	SC								
	PO								

mg/kg		Mouse	Rat	Guinea Pig	Rabbit	Cat	Dog	Monkey	
EEG (Desynchroni-zation)	IV								
	IP								
	IM								
	SC	10 109							
	PO								
Reverse Adrenergic Action of Guanethidine	IV					0.48 285			
	IP								
	IM								
	SC								
	PO								
	IV								
	IP								
	IM								
	SC								
	PO								
	IV								
	IP								
	IM								
	SC								
	PO								

IN VITRO

mg %	Cardiac	Vascular	Gut	Uterine	Visceral	Skeletal		
Rabbit		*0.004	0.1					

*Total mg

DIALLYLBARBITURIC ACID

(Dial, Allobarbital, Malilum)

mg/kg		Mouse	Rat	Guinea Pig	Rabbit	Cat	Dog	Monkey	
Lethal Dose Y$-$LD$_{50}$ Z$-$MLD	IV				70 [109]				
	IP				Z 100 [128]	100 [290]			
	IM								
	SC	Y 110 [68]			100 [109]				
	PO			30 [76]	Z 125 [128]				
Anesthetic	IV				50	36 [291]			
	IP					70 [292]			
	IM								
	SC		60 [66]						
	PO								
	IV								
	IP								
	IM								
	SC								
	PO								
	IV								
	IP								
	IM								
	SC								
	PO								

IN VITRO

mg %	Cardiac	Vascular	Gut	Uterine	Visceral	Skeletal		

DIAZEPAM

(Valium)

mg/kg		Mouse	Rat	Guinea Pig	Rabbit	Cat	Dog	Monkey	
Lethal Dose Y–LD$_{50}$ Z–MLD	IV				Y8.8 [845]				
	IP	Y220 [1145]							
	IM								
	SC								
	PO	Y970 [1145]							
Skeletal Muscle Relaxant	IV				6.6 [845]	3 [845]			
	IP								
	IM								
	SC								
	PO	25 [977]							
EEG and ECP	IV				2 [1223]	10 [843]			
	IP		5 [1069]						
	IM							1 [1195]	
	SC								
	PO								
Behavioral	IV					5 [1148]	1 [1107]		
	IP	6 [1115]	10 [977]			4 [1147]			
	IM								
	SC		1 [1129]						
	PO		152 [977]			6 [1108]	1 [977]		
Cardiovascular	IV					0.1 [875]	0.3 [1107]		
	IP		2 [1243]						
	IM								
	SC								
	PO								
Ataxic	IV								
	IP								
	IM								
	SC								
	PO	57 [881]							
Anticonvulsant	IV					0.25 [1117]			
	IP	10 [1148]				0.6 [1149]			
	IM							1 [1096]	
	SC	6.4 [920]							
	PO	18.7 [881]	2 [1072]			5 [920]			

DIBOZANE
(McN-181)

mg/kg		Mouse	Rat	Guinea Pig	Rabbit	Cat	Dog	Monkey	
Lethal Dose Y−LD$_{50}$ Z−MLD	IV				Y43 [293]		60 [293]		
	IP	Y260 [293]							
	IM								
	SC								
	PO								
Adrenolytic	IV						2 [294]		
	IP								
	IM								
	SC								
	PO						1 [293]		
Sympatholytic	IV						3 [295]		
	IP								
	IM								
	SC								
	PO								
	IV								
	IP								
	IM								
	SC								
	PO								

IN VITRO

mg %	Cardiac	Vascular	Gut	Uterine	Visceral	Skeletal		
Adrenolytic					0.003			

DICHLOROISOPROTERENOL

(DCI)

mg/kg		Mouse	Rat	Guinea Pig	Rabbit	Cat	Dog	Monkey	
Lethal Dose	IV	Y48 [296]							
Y—LD$_{50}$	IP	Y132 [296]							
Z—MLD	IM								
	SC								
	PO								
Cardiovascular	IV				10	10 [296]	10 [299]		
	IP								
	IM								
	SC								
	PO								
Adrenolytic (β-Block)	IV		0.1 [297]		4 [298]	4 [298]	2 [300]		
	IP								
	IM								
	SC								
	PO								
CNS	IV				4 [995]	7 [994]			
	IP								
	IM								
	SC								
	PO								

IN VITRO

mg %	Cardiac	Vascular	Gut	Uterine	Visceral	Skeletal		
Adrenolytic	0.04 [301]			1.0 [296]				
Sympathomimetic	0.65 [302]							

DIGITOXIN

(Digitaline, Crystodigin, Cardigin)

mg/kg		Mouse	Rat	Guinea Pig	Rabbit	Cat	Dog	Monkey	
Lethal Dose Y−LD_{50} Z−MLD	IV		12.2 [74]	Z1.2 [922]	3 [303]	0.35 [303]	Z0.65 [897]		
	IP								
	IM								
	SC	Y22.2 [922]	Y16.4 [922]			0.35 [303]	0.5 [303]		
	PO	Y32.7 [922]	Y23.8 [922]	Y>100 [922]	100 [303]	0.25			
Cardiovascular	IV						0.15		
	IP								
	IM								
	SC						0.15		
	PO								
	IV								
	IP								
	IM								
	SC								
	PO								
	IV								
	IP								
	IM								
	SC								
	PO								

IN VITRO

mg %	Cardiac	Vascular	Gut	Uterine	Visceral	Skeletal		

mg/kg		Mouse	Rat	Guinea Pig	Rabbit	Cat	Dog	Monkey	
Lethal Dose Y−LD$_{50}$ Z−MLD	IV	20 [149]			3.56 [149]	0.35 [149]	0.3 [149]		
	IP		> 10 [149]						
	IM			0.6 [149]					
	SC			0.45 [149]					
	PO			1.8 [149]			0.3 [149]		
Cardiac Arrhythmia	IV					0.15 [149]	0.2 [149]		
	IP								
	IM								
	SC								
	PO								
	IV								
	IP								
	IM								
	SC								
	PO								
	IV								
	IP								
	IM								
	SC								
	PO								

IN VITRO

mg %	Cardiac	Vascular	Gut	Uterine	Visceral	Skeletal		

DIHYDROERGOTAMINE

(D H E-45)

mg/kg		Mouse	Rat	Guinea Pig	Rabbit	Cat	Dog	Monkey	
Lethal Dose $Y-LD_{50}$ $Z-MLD$	IV	Y118 [304]	Y110 [304]		Y25 [304]				
	IP								
	IM								
	SC					Y68 [304]			
	PO								
Adrenolytic	IV		0.5 [218]		1.0 [305]		10		
	IP								
	IM								
	SC	3.16 [1212]							
	PO								
Sympatho-mimetic	IV						0.1 [306]		
	IP								
	IM								
	SC								
	PO								
Antiarrhythmic	IV						0.1 [1181]		
	IP								
	IM								
	SC								
	PO								

IN VITRO

mg %	Cardiac	Vascular	Gut	Uterine	Visceral	Skeletal		
Adrenolytic					0.02			

92

DIHYDROMORPHINONE

(Dilaudid, Laudicon, Hymorphan)

mg/kg		Mouse	Rat	Guinea Pig	Rabbit	Cat	Dog	Monkey	
Lethal Dose Y–LD$_{50}$ Z–MLD	IV	Y88 [307]							
	IP								
	IM								
	SC	Y84 [308]							
	PO								
Anesthetic	IV						3.5 [557]		
	IP								
	IM								
	SC						7.5 [557]		
	PO								
Analgetic	IV		1.32 [269]						
	IP	0.25 [309]	1.7 [269]	3.1 [309]					
	IM					0.26 [310]			
	SC		0.9 [269]				2		
	PO		18 [269]						
Behavioral	IV						10		
	IP		7.1 [310]						
	IM								
	SC								
	PO								
Catatonic	IV								
	IP		4 [269]						
	IM								
	SC								
	PO								
	IV								
	IP								
	IM								
	SC								
	PO								

DIISOPROPYL FLUOROPHOSPHATE

(DFP, Floropryl, Diflupyl)

mg/kg		Mouse	Rat	Guinea Pig	Rabbit	Cat	Dog	Monkey	
Lethal Dose Y−LD$_{50}$ Z−MLD	IV				Y0.34 [311]	Y1.63 [311]	Y3.43 [311]	Y0.25 [311]	
	IP								
	IM		Y1.82 [311]						
	SC	Y3.71 [311]	Y3.0 [311]		Y1.0 [311]		Y3.0 [311]		
	PO	Y36.8 [311]	Y6.0 [311]		Y9.78 [311]				
Anticholine-esterase	IV								
	IP								
	IM		1 [312]				1 [312]	0.20 [312]	
	SC								
	PO							0.50 [312]	
Sedative	IV								
	IP								
	IM		1 [312]				2 [312]		
	SC	2.5 [996]							
	PO								
Behavioral	IV								
	IP								
	IM								
	SC		1 [1140]						
	PO								

IN VITRO

mg %	Cardiac	Vascular	Gut	Uterine	Visceral	Skeletal		

mg/kg		Mouse	Rat	Guinea Pig	Rabbit	Cat	Dog	Monkey	
Lethal Dose Y−LD$_{50}$ Z−MLD	IV		Y26.8 [93]				Y45 [93]		
	IP								
	IM								
	SC								
	PO		Y618.2 [93]	Y888 [93]					
Antihistaminic	IV								
	IP								
	IM								
	SC								
	PO			0.06 [93]					
Cardiovascular	IV						9 [93]		
	IP								
	IM								
	SC								
	PO								
	IV								
	IP								
	IM								
	SC								
	PO								

IN VITRO

mg %	Cardiac	Vascular	Gut	Uterine	Visceral	Skeletal		
Antihistaminic			0.0007 [93]					
Anticholinergic			0.4 [93]					

2,4-DINITROPHENOL

(α-Dinitrophenol, Aldifen)

mg/kg		Mouse	Rat	Guinea Pig	Rabbit	Cat	Dog	Monkey	
Lethal Dose Y−LD$_{50}$ Z−MLD	IV						Y30 [315]		
	IP				100 [318]				
	IM						Y20 [315]		
	SC		Y25 [315]		30 [315]		Y22 [315]		
	PO		Y30 [316]		Y200 [318]		Y25 [315]		
Hyperthermic	IV						5 [319]		
	IP				10 [120]				
	IM						5 [319]		
	SC		10 [317]		20 [319]		5 [319]		
	PO						5 [319]		
Respiratory	IV						20 [319]		
	IP								
	IM				20 [319]				
	SC				20 [311]				
	PO								
	IV								
	IP								
	IM								
	SC								
	PO								

IN VITRO

mg %	Cardiac	Vascular	Gut	Uterine	Visceral	Skeletal		

DIPHENHYDRAMINE

(Benadryl, Dimedrol, Amidryl)

mg/kg		Mouse	Rat	Guinea Pig	Rabbit	Cat	Dog	Monkey	
Lethal Dose Y—LD$_{50}$ Z—MLD	IV	Y31	Y42 [321]		Y10 [321]		Y24 [321]		
	IP	Y84 [320]	Y82 [324]	Y75 [324]					
	IM								
	SC	Y127 [321]	Y475 [321]	40.2 [221]					
	PO	Y164 [321]	Y500 [325]	284 [221]					
Antihistaminic	IV			23 [221]		1.8 [97]	1.8 [97]		
	IP			12.5					
	IM					1.8 [97]	1.8 [97]		
	SC		10 [997]	5					
	PO						2.2 [97]		
Anticonvulsant	IV								
	IP	30 [251]	2 [930]						
	IM	15.7 [140]							
	SC								
	PO	30 [322]	25 [326]						
CNS	IV				15 [108]	1.5 [1206]			
	IP								
	IM								
	SC								
	PO								
Behavioral	IV								
	IP	40 [323]							
	IM								
	SC								
	PO	50 [935]							
Cholinolytic	IV				8 [839]				
	IP								
	IM								
	SC	22 [839]							
	PO								

97

DMPP

(Dimethylphenylpiperazine)

mg/kg		Mouse	Rat	Guinea Pig	Rabbit	Cat	Dog	Monkey	
Lethal Dose Y−LD$_{50}$ Z−MLD	IV				1 [314]		20 [313]		
	IP	Y40 [313]							
	IM	Y27.5 [314]							
	SC								
	PO	Y365 [313]	Y2000 [313]						
Ganglionic Stimulant	IV					0.2 [314]	0.15 [314]		
	IP								
	IM		0.5 [1167]						
	SC								
	PO								
Cardiovascular	IV				20 [313]	0.25 [313]	2 [313]		
	IP								
	IM								
	SC								
	PO								
	IV								
	IP								
	IM								
	SC								
	PO								

IN VITRO

mg %	Cardiac	Vascular	Gut	Uterine	Visceral	Skeletal		
Langendorff	*0.025 [314]							
Guinea Pig			0.4 [314]					

*Total mg

DOPA
(Dihydroxyphenylalanine)

mg/kg		Mouse	Rat	Guinea Pig	Rabbit	Cat	Dog	Monkey	
Lethal Dose Y$-$LD$_{50}$ Z$-$MLD	IV								
	IP		*10 328						
	IM								
	SC								
	PO								
Behavioral	IV				25 14				
	IP	750 327	20 329						
	IM								
	SC		200 942						
	PO								
Cardiovascular	IV		12 328						
	IP		12 328						
	IM								
	SC								
	PO								
CNS	IV		50 1226		50 1102	20 1098	1.3 1225		
	IP								
	IM								
	SC								
	PO								

*Total dose

IN VITRO

mg %	Cardiac	Vascular	Gut	Uterine	Visceral	Skeletal		

DOPAMINE

(3-hydroxytyramine)

mg/kg		Mouse	Rat	Guinea Pig	Rabbit	Cat	Dog	Monkey	
Lethal Dose Y—LD$_{50}$ Z—MLD	IV								
	IP								
	IM								
	SC								
	PO								
Cardiovascular	IV			*0.08 330	*0.8 330	*0.16 330	0.15 330		
	IP								
	IM								
	SC								
	PO								
EEG (desynchroni-zation)	IV				15 331				
	IP								
	IM								
	SC								
	PO								
Neuromuscular Block	IV					5 1132			
	IP								
	IM								
	SC								
	PO								
CNS	IV						0.3 1225		
	IP								
	IM								
	SC								
	PO								
Decrease Adrenal Ascorbic Acid	IV								
	IP								
	IM								
	SC		10 857						
	PO								

*Total dose

mg/kg		Mouse	Rat	Guinea Pig	Rabbit	Cat	Dog	Monkey	
	IV								
	IP								
	IM								
	SC								
	PO								
	IV								
	IP								
	IM								
	SC								
	PO								
	IV								
	IP								
	IM								
	SC								
	PO								
	IV								
	IP								
	IM								
	SC								
	PO								

IN VITRO

mg %	Cardiac	Vascular	Gut	Uterine	Visceral	Skeletal		
Rabbit	0.16 [266]	100 [330]	0.024 [266]					
Cat	*5 [266]		0.164 [266]	0.26 [266]				
Hind Limb (Perfusion)		*0.64						

*Total mg

EDROPHONIUM

(Tensilon, RO2-3198)

mg/kg		Mouse	Rat	Guinea Pig	Rabbit	Cat	Dog	Monkey	
Lethal Dose $Y-LD_{50}$ $Z-MLD$	IV	Y9 [210]			Y28.5 [210]		Y15 [250]		
	IP	Y37 [210]							
	IM								
	SC	Y130 [210]							
	PO	Y600 [210]							
Curare Antagonist	IV					0.4	0.4		
	IP								
	IM								
	SC		2.5						
	PO								
Muscle Relaxant	IV					0.5	0.5		
	IP								
	IM								
	SC								
	PO								
	IV								
	IP								
	IM								
	SC								
	PO								

IN VITRO

mg %	Cardiac	Vascular	Gut	Uterine	Visceral	Skeletal		

EPHEDRINE

(Ephedral, Sanedrine, Biophedrin)

mg/kg		Mouse	Rat	Guinea Pig	Rabbit	Cat	Dog	Monkey	
Lethal Dose $Y-LD_{50}$ $Z-MLD$	IV	200 [6]	Z137 [334]		Z60 [6]	Z60 [6]	Z72.5 [333]		
	IP	Z400 [332]	800 [335]		Z355 [334]				
	IM				Z340 [333]				
	SC	500 [333]	Y650	400 [6]	Z360 [333]		Z220 [333]		
	PO	Y1550 [960]	Z160 [335]		Z590 [334]				
Behavioral	IV							15	
	IP	1.25 [177]							
	IM								
	SC	10 [940]							
	PO	100 [960]	100 [336]				0.06 [337]		
Cardiovascular	IV		1	1	1	1	0.5		
	IP								
	IM								
	SC								
	PO								
CNS Stimulant	IV						2.5		
	IP						3.3 [97]		
	IM								
	SC						2.5		
	PO						*20 [97]		
Antagonize Adrenolytic Action of Bretylium	IV					0.35 [153]			
	IP								
	IM								
	SC								
	PO								
Antagonize Reserpine	IV								
	IP	20 [78]							
	IM								
	SC								
	PO						2 [1168]		

*Total mg

103

EPHEDRINE (continued)

mg/kg		Mouse	Rat	Guinea Pig	Rabbit	Cat	Dog	Monkey	
Increase Rate of Catechol Amine Disappearance	IV								
	IP	50 338							
	IM								
	SC								
	PO								
Hyperthermic	IV								
	IP								
	IM								
	SC		60 259						
	PO								
	IV								
	IP								
	IM								
	SC								
	PO								
	IV								
	IP								
	IM								
	SC								
	PO								

IN VITRO

mg %	Cardiac	Vascular	Gut	Uterine	Visceral	Skeletal		
Rabbit			2 1157					
Rat			0.8 92	0.2 1157				
Guinea Pig			0.3 92					
Rabbit Ear		*0.016 339						

*Total mg

mg/kg		Mouse	Rat	Guinea Pig	Rabbit	Cat	Dog	Monkey	
Lethal Dose $Y-LD_{50}$ $Z-MLD$	IV	Y0.5 896	Y0.98	0.15 341	0.2 341	0.7 341	0.15 341		
	IP	Y4 340	10 343						
	IM		Y3.5 7						
	SC	Y1.47 341	Y5.0 341	1.5 341	15 341	20 341	5.5 341		
	PO	Y50	30 341		30 341				
Cardiovascular	IV	0.002 1197	0.002 855	0.003	0.003	0.003	0.003	0.001 1079	
	IP								
	IM						0.05		
	SC		1 862				0.05		
	PO								
Behavioral	IV						0.05 99		
	IP	2.5 177	1 344						
	IM								
	SC	2 940							
	PO								
CNS	IV				0.01 345	0.15 998			
	IP								
	IM								
	SC								
	PO								
Barbiturate Sleep Potentiation	IV								
	IP	2 342							
	IM	0.4 7							
	SC								
	PO								
Antagonize Reserpine Ptosis	IV								
	IP	1 78							
	IM								
	SC								
	PO								

EPINEPHRINE (continued)

mg/kg		Mouse	Rat	Guinea Pig	Rabbit	Cat	Dog	Monkey	
Diuretic	IV								
	IP								
	IM								
	SC		0.5 151				1 885		
	PO								
EEG	IV				0.004 827	0.004 827			
	IP								
	IM								
	SC								
	PO								
Metabolic	IV						0.022 865		
	IP		0.05 1082						
	IM								
	SC	0.1 1200	0.2 864		0.15 863				
	PO								
Bronchiole dilation	IV								
	IP								
	IM								
	SC			0.05 1081					
	PO								

IN VITRO

mg %	Cardiac	Vascular	Gut	Uterine	Visceral	Skeletal	Trachea	
Sympathomimetic	0.01	0.003	0.01	0.02	0.01		0.006 1157	
Langendorff	*0.1							
Antiserotonergic			0.002 92					

*Total mg

mg/kg		Mouse	Rat	Guinea Pig	Rabbit	Cat	Dog	Monkey	
Lethal Dose Y—LD$_{50}$ Z—MLD	IV	145 [346]		80 [346]	Z7.5				
	IP								
	IM								
	SC		0.5 [346]						
	PO								
Oxytocic	IV						*0.35 [97]		
	IP								
	IM						*0.35 [97]		
	SC		500 [257]						
	PO								
Antagonize Epinephrine Toxicity	IV		0.085						
	IP								
	IM								
	SC								
	PO								
	IV								
	IP								
	IM								
	SC								
	PO								

*Total dose

IN VITRO

mg %	Cardiac	Vascular	Gut	Uterine	Visceral	Skeletal		
Oxytocic				50 [347]				

ERGOTAMINE

(Gynergen, Femergin, Ergomar)

mg/kg		Mouse	Rat	Guinea Pig	Rabbit	Cat	Dog	Monkey	
Lethal Dose Y−LD$_{50}$ Z−MLD	IV	Y52 [348]	Y62 [304]	36 [351]	Y3.55 [352]				
	IP								
	IM								
	SC		Z125 [349]			Y11 [352]			
	PO								
Adrenolytic	IV				0.15 [352]	1	8 [354]		
	IP								
	IM							ı	
	SC								
	PO								
CNS	IV					0.1 [353]			
	IP								
	IM								
	SC		5 [350]						
	PO								
	IV								
	IP								
	IM								
	SC								
	PO								

IN VITRO

mg %	Cardiac	Vascular	Gut	Uterine	Visceral	Skeletal		
Rabbit				0.5 [352]				
Guinea Pig				0.002 [352]				

mg/kg		Mouse	Rat	Guinea Pig	Rabbit	Cat	Dog	Monkey	
Lethal Dose Y–LD$_{50}$ Z–MLD	IV				Ẏ0.25 [346]	Y0.2 [346]	Y0.06 [346]	Y4 [346]	
	IP	Y10 [346]	Y0.4 [346]	Y0.35 [346]					
	IM		Y5 [346]						
	SC	Y16 [346]	Y2.5 [346]	0.25 [346]	0.75 [346]				
	PO	Y8 [346]	Y2.5 [346]						
Decreased Mitotic Index of Mucosal Epithelium	IV						1.0 [355]		
	IP								
	IM								
	SC								
	PO								
	IV								
	IP								
	IM								
	SC								
	PO								
	IV								
	IP								
	IM								
	SC								
	PO								

IN VITRO

mg %	Cardiac	Vascular	Gut	Uterine	Visceral	Skeletal		
Rabbit			0.004 [356]					

GALLAMINE

(Flaxedil, Relaxan, Tricuran)

mg/kg		Mouse	Rat	Guinea Pig	Rabbit	Cat	Dog	Monkey	
Lethal Dose $Y-LD_{50}$ $Z-MLD$	IV	Y4.3	Y5.5 [361]		Y0.65 [361]		Y0.8 [361]		
	IP	Y9.6 [1143]							
	IM				Y2.5 [361]				
	SC	Y17.4 [360]	Y25 [361]		Y3.0 [361]				
	PO	Y425 [361]			Y100 [361]				
Neuromuscular Block	IV		0.01 [1143]		0.6 [88]	5 [362]	0.4 [361]		
	IP								
	IM				0.75 [361]				
	SC				1.5 [361]				
	PO								
CNS	IV		2 [1000]			1 [1000]			
	IP								
	IM								
	SC								
	PO								
	IV								
	IP								
	IM								
	SC								
	PO								

IN VITRO

mg %	Cardiac	Vascular	Gut	Uterine	Visceral	Skeletal		
Rat						0.25 [1157]		

GAMMA-AMINOBUTYRIC ACID

(GABA)

mg/kg		Mouse	Rat	Guinea Pig	Rabbit	Cat	Dog	Monkey	
Lethal Dose Y−LD$_{50}$ Z−MLD	IV								
	IP								
	IM								
	SC								
	PO								
Cardiovascular	IV				3.0 [208]	10 [208]	3.0 [208]		
	IP								
	IM								
	SC								
	PO								
CNS (Inhibition)	IV					0.1 [357]	100 [358]		
	IP								
	IM								
	SC	2500 [999]							
	PO								
Behavioral	IV	1000 [359]							
	IP								
	IM								
	SC								
	PO	400 [359]							
	IV								
	IP								
	IM								
	SC								
	PO								
	IV								
	IP								
	IM								
	SC								
	PO								

111

GUANETHIDINE

(Ismelin, SU-5864)

mg/kg		Mouse	Rat	Guinea Pig	Rabbit	Cat	Dog	Monkey	
Lethal Dose Y−LD$_{50}$ Z−MLD	IV	Y22 [93]	Y23 [363]		50	50			
	IP								
	IM								
	SC								
	PO		Y1000 [363]						
Autonomic Effects	IV				3	15 [363]	15		
	IP	2.5 [1243]		100 [1219]		15 [367]			
	IM								
	SC					7.5 [171]			
	PO					15 [171]	35 [93]		
Catechol Amine Depletion	IV		5 [150]		12.5 [366]	15 [91]			
	IP	10 [861]	8 [364]						
	IM		25 [150]						
	SC		15 [365]			15 [366]			
	PO								
	IV								
	IP								
	IM								
	SC								
	PO								

IN VITRO

mg %	Cardiac	Vascular	Gut	Uterine	Visceral	Skeletal		
Finkleman [812]			0.4 [365]					

HARMALINE

(3,4-dihydroharmine)

mg/kg		Mouse	Rat	Guinea Pig	Rabbit	Cat	Dog	Monkey	
Lethal Dose $Y-LD_{50}$ $Z-MLD$	IV				20 [1105]				
	IP								
	IM								
	SC	Y120 [115]	Z120 [368]	Z100 [368]	Z100 [368]	Z100 [368]	33.3 [368]		
	PO								
Cardiovascular and Uterine	IV				10 [371]	1 [368]	5		
	IP								
	IM								
	SC								
	PO								
Behavioral	IV								
	IP	8 [992]	5 [370]						
	IM								
	SC		2.5						
	PO								
Ataxic	IV				5 [1105]				
	IP	15 [369]	10						
	IM								
	SC			10 [368]					
	PO								
Spinal Reflex Depressant	IV					5 [372]			
	IP								
	IM								
	SC								
	PO								
Tremor	IV				3 [1105]	5 [1244]			
	IP		15 [1105]						
	IM								
	SC								
	PO								

HARMINE

(Banisterine, Yageine, Telepathine)

mg/kg		Mouse	Rat	Guinea Pig	Rabbit	Cat	Dog	Monkey	
Lethal Dose Y—LD$_{50}$ Z—MLD	IV				60 $_{1105}$				
	IP								
	IM								
	SC	300 $_{373}$	Z 200 $_{374}$	100 $_{375}$	200 $_{375}$	Z 200 $_{373}$		Z 30 $_{373}$	
	PO								
Cardiovascular	IV				10 $_{374}$	4 $_{374}$	5		
	IP								
	IM								
	SC								
	PO								
Tremor	IV				3 $_{1105}$				
	IP	15 $_{369}$	15 $_{1105}$						
	IM	10 $_{175}$							
	SC								
	PO								
Behavioral	IV								
	IP								
	IM	1 $_{175}$							
	SC								
	PO								
Ganglionic Block	IV					25 $_{376}$	15 $_{376}$		
	IP								
	IM								
	SC								
	PO								
EEG	IV					5 $_{842}$			
	IP								
	IM								
	SC								
	PO								

mg/kg		Mouse	Rat	Guinea Pig	Rabbit	Cat	Dog	Monkey	
Lethal Dose Y−LD$_{50}$ Z−MLD	IV				1.2 [1110]	1 [378]	2.5 [1110]		
	IP	Y0.064 [377]	Y0.45 [1110]	0.75 [1110]					
	IM								
	SC								
	PO								
Parasympatho-lytic	IV				5.9 [377]		0.013 [377]		
	IP								
	IM								
	SC								
	PO								
CNS	IV					3.5 [379]	10 [1078]		
	IP								
	IM								
	SC								
	PO								
Neuromuscular block	IV				1.8 [872]				
	IP								
	IM								
	SC								
	PO								

IN VITRO

mg %	Cardiac	Vascular	Gut	Uterine	Visceral	Skeletal		
Guinea Pig						20 [100]		
Rat						20		
Rabbit	4 [100]			2.4 [100]				
Cat	50 [100]							

HEPARIN

(Panheparin, Liquemin, Pularin)

mg/kg		Mouse	Rat	Guinea Pig	Rabbit	Cat	Dog	Monkey	
Lethal Dose Y—LD$_{50}$ Z—MLD	IV	Y1780 [380]							
	IP								
	IM								
	SC								
	PO								
Anticoagulant	IV		10 [381]		5 [383]	5 [385]	8 [209]	2	
	IP								
	IM								
	SC								
	PO								
Increased Lipoproeteinase Activity	IV		6 [382]		1.5 [384]				
	IP								
	IM								
	SC								
	PO								
	IV								
	IP								
	IM								
	SC								
	PO								

IN VITRO

mg %	Cardiac	Vascular	Gut	Uterine	Visceral	Skeletal		

HEXAMETHONIUM

(C6, Hexameton, Bistrium)

mg/kg		Mouse	Rat	Guinea Pig	Rabbit	Cat	Dog	Monkey	
Lethal Dose Y−LD$_{50}$ Z−MLD	IV	Y21 214							
	IP	Y42 214							
	IM								
	SC								
	PO	Y484 214							
Ganglionic Block	IV		20 386	5	10	10	10		
	IP		2.8 387	10 1219					
	IM								
	SC								
	PO		100 387						
CNS	IV								
	IP	5 350							
	IM								
	SC		2 350						
	PO								
Behavioral	IV								
	IP			5 1109					
	IM								
	SC			10 1092					
	PO	40 935							

IN VITRO

mg %	Cardiac	Vascular	Gut	Uterine	Visceral	Skeletal		
Rat			0.24 388			1.5 1157		
Rabbit	10		5					
Guinea Pig			2 1157					

HEXOBARBITAL

(Evipan, Cyclonal, Privenal)

mg/kg		Mouse	Rat	Guinea Pig	Rabbit	Cat	Dog	Monkey	
Lethal Dose $Y-LD_{50}$ $Z-MLD$	IV	190 [389]			Y80 [66]	100 [66]	100 [66]		
	IP	Y340 [390]	Y280 [393]	100 [66]	Z225* [393]				
	IM								
	SC	250 [66]	404 [66]						
	PO	Y468 [391]	Y468		Z1200 [394]	400 [66]			
Anesthetic	IV	47 [392]	25 [1076]		25	25 [66]	30 [66]		
	IP	75	75 [393]		40 [395]	40 [395]			
	IM								
	SC	150 [66]	90 [66]						
	PO	150 [66]				100 [66]			
Increased Brain Serotonin	IV								
	IP		100 [31]						
	IM								
	SC								
	PO								
Behavioral	IV								
	IP	26 [204]						20 [1230]	
	IM								
	SC								
	PO								
Decreased Hippocampal Seizure	IV					20 [396]			
	IP								
	IM								
	SC								
	PO								
Decreased Spinal Reflexes	IV		5 [1000]			5 [1000]			
	IP								
	IM								
	SC								
	PO								

mg/kg		Mouse	Rat	Guinea Pig	Rabbit	Cat	Dog	Monkey	
Lethal Dose $Y-LD_{50}$ $Z-MLD$	IV	Y10.5 [111]							
	IP	Y55 [111]							
	IM								
	SC	Y360 [111]							
	PO	Y600 [111]							
Anticholinergic	IV					4 [111]	5 [111]		
	IP								
	IM								
	SC								
	PO								
Antispasmotic	IV						0.04 [111]		
	IP								
	IM								
	SC								
	PO								
	IV								
	IP								
	IM								
	SC								
	PO								

IN VITRO

mg %	Cardiac	Vascular	Gut	Uterine	Visceral	Skeletal		

119

HISTAMINE

(Eramin, Ergamine, Ergotidine)

mg/kg		Mouse	Rat	Guinea Pig	Rabbit	Cat	Dog	Monkey	
Lethal Dose Y-LD$_{50}$ Z-MLD	IV			Y0.18 [398]	0.1 [109]		30	50 [109]	
	IP			33 [399]			-		
	IM								
	SC	2500 [195]		7 [399]	13.5 [399]				
	PO			300 [400]					
Cardiovascular	IV		0.01 [855]	0.1	0.15	0.005	0.005		
	IP								
	IM								
	SC						1		
	PO								
Increase Stomach HCl	IV								
	IP								
	IM								
	SC						*0.1		
	PO		25 [397]				0.5 [397]		
Behavioral	IV								
	IP								
	IM								
	SC	10 [935]							
	PO								

*Total dose

IN VITRO

mg %	Cardiac	Vascular	Gut	Uterine	Visceral	Skeletal	Trachea	
Guinea Pig			0.005	0.005			0.06 [1157]	
Rabbit	0.1	0.003 [1157]		0.5				
Rat			0.3 [1157]	3 [1157]				

HOMATROPINE

(Malcotran, Mesopin, Novatropine)

mg/kg		Mouse	Rat	Guinea Pig	Rabbit	Cat	Dog	Monkey	
Lethal Dose Y$-$LD$_{50}$ Z$-$MLD	IV								
	IP	Y60 [101]	Y82 [101]	Y120 [101]					
	IM								
	SC	Y650 [101]	Y800 [101]						
	PO	Y1400 [101]	Y1200 [101]	Y1000 [101]					
Anticholinergic	IV								
	IP								
	IM				0.16 [101]				
	SC	0.13 [101]	27 [101]						
	PO	12 [101]	18 [101]						
Ganglionic Block	IV					1.0 [101]			
	IP								
	IM								
	SC								
	PO								
	IV								
	IP								
	IM								
	SC								
	PO								

IN VITRO

mg %	Cardiac	Vascular	Gut	Uterine	Visceral	Skeletal		
Rabbit			0.01					

HORDENINE

(Anhaline)

mg/kg		Mouse	Rat	Guinea Pig	Rabbit	Cat	Dog	Monkey	
Lethal Dose Y−LD$_{50}$ Z−MLD	IV			300 [401]	275 [109]		275 [109]		
	IP								
	IM								
	SC		1000 [401]	2000 [401]					
	PO						2000 [109]		
Cardiovascular	IV					*2 [402]			
	IP								
	IM								
	SC								
	PO								
Block Diarrhea	IV								
	IP								
	IM								
	SC						35 [274]		
	PO								
	IV								
	IP								
	IM								
	SC								
	PO								

*Total dose

IN VITRO

mg %	Cardiac	Vascular	Gut	Uterine	Visceral	Skeletal		
Stimulation			0.8 [402]	0.8 [402]				

1-HYDRAZINOPHTHALAZINE

(Apresoline, Hydralazine)

mg/kg		Mouse	Rat	Guinea Pig	Rabbit	Cat	Dog	Monkey	
Lethal Dose $Y-LD_{50}$ $Z-MLD$	IV		34 [403]				64 [817]		
	IP	Y83 [817]							
	IM								
	SC								
	PO		173 [93]						
Cardiovascular	IV		1.0 [403]	1.0 [403]		1.0 [403]	1.0 [403]		
	IP		2.6 [404]						
	IM								
	SC		0.57 [916]						
	PO								
Adrenolytic	IV					1.0 [405]	8.0 [817]		
	IP								
	IM								
	SC								
	PO								
Cardiovascular Reflex	IV						1 [1177]		
	IP								
	IM								
	SC								
	PO								

IN VITRO

mg %	Cardiac	Vascular	Gut	Uterine	Visceral	Skeletal		
Spasmogenic			10 [403]					

HYDROCHLOROTHIAZIDE

(Esidrex, Hydro-Diuril, Oretic)

mg/kg		Mouse	Rat	Guinea Pig	Rabbit	Cat	Dog	Monkey	
Lethal Dose Y—LD$_{50}$ Z—MLD	IV	Y884 [58]			Y461 [58]		Y250 [58]		
	IP	Y578 [58]	Y234 [58]						
	IM								
	SC	Y1470 [58]	Y1270 [58]						
	PO	Y3080 [58]	Y6190 [58]						
Diuretic	IV						0.5 [58]		
	IP		15 [58]						
	IM						10 [1077]		
	SC								
	PO		15 [58]				0.25 [58]	10 [58]	
	IV								
	IP								
	IM								
	SC								
	PO								
	IV								
	IP								
	IM								
	SC								
	PO								

IN VITRO

mg %	Cardiac	Vascular	Gut	Uterine	Visceral	Skeletal		

p-HYDROXY-α-(METHYLAMINOMETHYL) BENZYL ALCOHOL

(Araleptin, Sympatol, Synephrin)

mg/kg		Mouse	Rat	Guinea Pig	Rabbit	Cat	Dog	Monkey	
Lethal Dose Y−LD$_{50}$ Z−MLD	IV								
	IP								
	IM								
	SC	750 [406]							
	PO								
Cardiovascular	IV					*0.7 [266]	0.25 [408]		
	IP								
	IM								
	SC								
	PO								
Decrease Catechol Amine Binding	IV								
	IP	40 [338]							
	IM								
	SC								
	PO								
Oxytocic	IV		2.5 [407]						
	IP								
	IM								
	SC								
	PO								
	IV								
	IP								
	IM								
	SC								
	PO								
	IV								
	IP								
	IM								
	SC								
	PO								

*Total dose

L-3-HYDROXY-N-METHYLMORPHINAN

(Levorphanol, Levo-Dromoran, Levorphan)

mg/kg		Mouse	Rat	Guinea Pig	Rabbit	Cat	Dog	Monkey	
Lethal Dose Y−LD$_{50}$ Z−MLD	IV	Y41.5 [210]			Y20 [210]				
	IP								
	IM								
	SC	Y187 [210]	.Y110 [210]						
	PO	Y285 [210]	Y150 [210]						
Analgetic	IV								
	IP								
	IM								
	SC		2.0 [435]				2		
	PO								
Respiratory	IV				0.5 [435]				
	IP								
	IM								
	SC								
	PO								
Antitussive	IV						2 [435]		
	IP								
	IM								
	SC								
	PO								
	IV								
	IP								
	IM								
	SC								
	PO								
	IV								
	IP								
	IM								
	SC								
	PO								

DL-3-HYDROXY-N-METHYLMORPHINAN

(Dromoran, Methorphinan, Racemorphan)

mg/kg		Mouse	Rat	Guinea Pig	Rabbit	Cat	Dog	Monkey	
Lethal Dose	IV	41 [409]			19 [409]				
Y—LD$_{50}$	IP	120 [409]							
Z—MLD	IM								
	SC	153 [409]	125 [409]						
	PO								
Analgetic	IV								
	IP								
	IM								
	SC		1.0 [409]						
	PO		10 [409]						
Respiratory Depressant	IV				2.0 [409]				
	IP								
	IM								
	SC								
	PO								
Increased Intestinal Motility	IV						2 [409]		
	IP								
	IM								
	SC								
	PO								
Cardiovascular	IV					4 [409]	4 [409]		
	IP								
	IM								
	SC								
	PO								
	IV								
	IP								
	IM								
	SC								
	PO								

5-HYDROXYTRYPTOPHAN

(5-HTP)

mg/kg		Mouse	Rat	Guinea Pig	Rabbit	Cat	Dog	Monkey	
Lethal Dose Y−LD$_{50}$ Z−MLD	IV								
	IP								
	IM								
	SC								
	PO								
Behavioral	IV	25 [286]	25 [411]						
	IP	100 [204]							
	IM								
	SC	10 [1001]	40 [286]						
	PO								
CNS	IV				65 [410]	100 [412]	50 [410]		
	IP	45 [410]	75 [410]						
	IM								
	SC								
	PO								
Gastrointestinal Stimulant	IV					60 [410]	60 [410]		
	IP	60 [410]	60 [410]						
	IM								
	SC								
	PO								
Cardiovascular	IV				87.5 [410]		30 [413]		
	IP								
	IM								
	SC								
	PO								
Anticonvulsant	IV								
	IP								
	IM								
	SC		30 [414]						
	PO								

mg/kg		Mouse	Rat	Guinea Pig	Rabbit	Cat	Dog	Monkey	
Decreased Motor Activity	IV					50 [410]	30 [413]		
	IP								
	IM								
	SC								
	PO								
EEG	IV				0.03 [827]	0.03 [827]			
	IP								
	IM								
	SC								
	PO								
Decrease Catecholamines	IV								
	IP	5 [861]							
	IM								
	SC								
	PO								
	IV								
	IP								
	IM								
	SC								
	PO								

IN VITRO

mg %	Cardiac	Vascular	Gut	Uterine	Visceral	Skeletal		

HYDROXYZINE

(Atarax, Placidol, Tran-Q)

mg/kg		Mouse	Rat	Guinea Pig	Rabbit	Cat	Dog	Monkey	
Lethal Dose Y−LD$_{50}$ Z−MLD	IV	137 [117]	Y45 [986]						
	IP	137 [117]	137 [117]						
	IM								
	SC								
	PO	515 [226]	Y1000 [986]						
Behavioral	IV							10 [418]	
	IP	70 [137]	20 [416]				0.1 [417]		
	IM	250 [175]							
	SC	100 [415]	25 [1002]						
	PO	50 [1002]	250 [1002]						
Tolerated	IV							12.5 [117]	
	IP								
	IM								
	SC								
	PO	490 [226]					20 [117]	87.5 [117]	
Barbiturate Sleep Potentiation	IV								
	IP								
	IM								
	SC	50 [142]		50 [142]	50 [142]				
	PO		50 [986]						
Analgetic	IV								
	IP	89 [1119]							
	IM								
	SC			50 [142]					
	PO			100 [142]					
EEG (Synchroni- zation)	IV				6 [108]				
	IP								
	IM								
	SC								
	PO								

mg/kg		Mouse	Rat	Guinea Pig	Rabbit	Cat	Dog	Monkey	
Cardiovascular	IV				1 [1002]	2 [1002]	7.5 [419]		
	IP								
	IM								
	SC		10 [986]						
	PO								
Antidiuretic	IV						5 [420]		
	IP								
	IM								
	SC								
	PO								
Increased EEG Arousal Threshold	IV				16 [831]				
	IP								
	IM								
	SC								
	PO								
	IV								
	IP								
	IM								
	SC								
	PO								

IN VITRO

mg %	Cardiac	Vascular	Gut	Uterine	Visceral	Skeletal		

131

ILIDAR

(Azepine, Azapetine, RO-2-3248)

mg/kg		Mouse	Rat	Guinea Pig	Rabbit	Cat	Dog	Monkey	
Lethal Dose $Y-LD_{50}$ $Z-MLD$	IV	Y27 [210]			Y28 [210]		Y50 [210]		
	IP	Y210 [210]							
	IM	Y600 [421]							
	SC	Y725 [210]							
	PO	Y460 [210]							
Adrenolytic (Cardiac)	IV						32 [422]		
	IP								
	IM								
	SC								
	PO								
Analgetic Hypothermic	IV								
	IP								
	IM								
	SC		100 [421]						
	PO								
Cardiovascular	IV						1 [421]		
	IP								
	IM								
	SC								
	PO						10 [421]		
Antifibrillatory	IV						3 [421]		
	IP								
	IM								
	SC								
	PO								
	IV								
	IP								
	IM								
	SC								
	PO								

IMIPRAMINE

(Tofranil, G22355, Imizin)

mg/kg		Mouse	Rat	Guinea Pig	Rabbit	Cat	Dog	Monkey	
Lethal Dose Y−LD$_{50}$ Z−MLD	IV	Y35 [235]	Y22 [235]		Y18 [235]				
	IP	Y115 [59]	Y79						
	IM								
	SC	Y189	Y250						
	PO	Y400 [235]	Y625 [235]						
Barbiturate Sleep Potentiation	IV						5 [425]		
	IP	50 [978]							
	IM								
	SC	50 [423]			50 [142]				
	PO			25 [105]					
CNS	IV	14 [838]			10 [235]	8 [1005]			
	IP	32 [949]	20 [59]			4 [1004]			
	IM								
	SC	50 [235]	50 [235]	50 [978]		20 [235]			
	PO								
Antagonize Reserpine	IV				15 [988]				
	IP	75 [264]	15 [810]						
	IM								
	SC								
	PO	100 [79]							
Cardiovascular	IV					1 [235]	4 [426]		
	IP								
	IM								
	SC								
	PO								
Decreased Motor Activity	IV								
	IP		40 [1003]	30 [978]					
	IM								
	SC	50 [105]				10 [424]			
	PO								

IMIPRAMINE (continued)

mg/kg		Mouse	Rat	Guinea Pig	Rabbit	Cat	Dog	Monkey	
EEG	IV				4.5 [831]	3 [1102]		7 [949]	
	IP								
	IM						10 [1006]		
	SC				20 [837]				
	PO								
Decreased Catachoamine Uptake	IV								
	IP	20 [910]				20 [91]			
	IM								
	SC								
	PO								
Serotonin and Catachoamine Potentiation	IV					2.4 [427]			
	IP								
	IM								
	SC								
	PO								
Behavioral	IV					5 [850]		3.5 [949]	
	IP	20 [874]	8 [848]			10 [1149]			
	IM								
	SC								
	PO	100 [935]	160 [949]					20 [949]	

IN VITRO

mg %	Cardiac	Vascular	Gut	Uterine	Visceral	Skeletal		
Anticholinergic			*0.16 [235]					
Antihistiminic		*0.006 [235]						
Anti-BaCl$_2$			*0.3 [235]					
Antiserotonergic			*0.004 [235]					

*Total mg

IPRONIAZID

(Iprazid, Marsilid, RO-2-4572)

mg/kg		Mouse	Rat	Guinea Pig	Rabbit	Cat	Dog	Monkey	
Lethal Dose Y−LD$_{50}$ Z−MLD	IV	Y725 [428]			Y150 [428]		140 [429]		
	IP	Y690 [428]							
	IM	Y683 [428]							
	SC	Y750 [428]							
	PO	Y968 [428]	Y383 [428]		Y150 [428]		140 [428]	640 [429]	
Monoamine Oxidase Inhibition	IV	100 [430]				100 [430]	65 [372]		
	IP	25 [429]	50 [429]						
	IM								
	SC	100 [430]	12 [868]		100 [430]	100 [430]			
	PO		100 [433]						
Increased Brain Serotonin and Norepinephrine	IV								
	IP	300 [431]	100 [148]						
	IM								
	SC		100 [434]		100				
	PO								
Barbiturate Sleep Potentiation	IV								
	IP	100 [411]							
	IM								
	SC	50 [142]		50 [142]	50 [142]				
	PO								
Cardiovascular	IV					8 [428]	163 [372]		
	IP								
	IM								
	SC								
	PO								
Behavioral	IV								
	IP	200 [874]	155 [848]						
	IM								
	SC	100 [432]	100 [370]				129 [955]		
	PO					2 [1007]			

IPRONIAZID (continued)

mg/kg		Mouse	Rat	Guinea Pig	Rabbit	Cat	Dog	Monkey	
Analgetic	IV								
	IP								
	IM								
	SC	100 1008		50 142					
	PO								
Ganglionic Block	IV					100 376			
	IP								
	IM								
	SC								
	PO								
Decreased Motor Activity	IV								
	IP	200 204							
	IM								
	SC	100 1008							
	PO								
	IV								
	IP								
	IM								
	SC								
	PO								

IN VITRO

mg %	Cardiac	Vascular	Gut	Uterine	Visceral	Skeletal		
Cat	10 429							

mg/kg		Mouse	Rat	Guinea Pig	Rabbit	Cat	Dog	Monkey	
Lethal Dose $Y-LD_{50}$ $Z-MLD$	IV								
	IP	Y110 [210]	Y199 [210]						
	IM								
	SC								
	PO	Y173 [210]	Y280 [115]				40 [429]	160 [429]	
Monoamine Oxidase Inhibition	IV								
	IP	0.75 [429]	2 [429]	*5 [1169]				20 [1170]	
	IM								
	SC								
	PO								
Reserpine Antagonist	IV								
	IP	5 [455]							
	IM								
	SC								
	PO	15 [455]							
Barbiturate Sleep Potentiation	IV								
	IP								
	IM								
	SC	25 [142]							
	PO			50 [142]					
Behavioral	IV								
	IP								
	IM								
	SC		1.2 [456]						
	PO								
CNS	IV					5 [1009]			
	IP		3 [1201]						
	IM								
	SC								
	PO								

*for 6 days

ISONIAZID

(Armazide, INH, Rimifon)

mg/kg		Mouse	Rat	Guinea Pig	Rabbit	Cat	Dog	Monkey	
Lethal Dose $Y-LD_{50}$ $Z-MLD$	IV	Y153 [428]			Y94 [428]		100 [428]		
	IP	Y132 [428]							
	IM	Y140 [428]							
	SC	Y160 [428]							
	PO	Y142 [428]	Y650 [115]		250 [428]		100 [428]		
Cardiovascular	IV					8 [428]			
	IP								
	IM								
	SC								
	PO								
Behavioral	IV								
	IP								
	IM								
	SC		100 [1010]						
	PO								
	IV								
	IP								
	IM								
	SC								
	PO								

IN VITRO

mg %	Cardiac	Vascular	Gut	Uterine	Visceral	Skeletal		

mg/kg		Mouse	Rat	Guinea Pig	Rabbit	Cat	Dog	Monkey	
Lethal Dose Y−LD$_{50}$ Z−MLD	IV	Y128 1084					Y50 1084		
	IP	Y300 111							
	IM								
	SC			Y0.32 1084					
	PO	Y450 111		Y270 1084					
Cardiovascular Sympatho-mimetic (Cardiovascular, Bronchodilator)	IV			0.01	0.002 298	0.005	0.005		
	IP								
	IM								
	SC		0.1 862	0.06 1084					
	PO			17 1084					
EEG (Desynchroni-zation)	IV				0.005 298	0.005 298	0.005 298		
	IP								
	IM								
	SC								
	PO								
Metabolic	IV						0.022 865		
	IP		0.05 1082						
	IM								
	SC		0.02 864		25 863				
	PO								

IN VITRO

mg %	Cardiac	Vascular	Gut	Uterine	Visceral	Skeletal	Trachea	
Langendorff	*0.001							
Guinea Pig						0.01	0.003 1157	
Rabbit	0.025	0.01 1157	0.01					
Rat				0.0003 1157				

*Total mg

LEVALLORPHAN

(Lorfan, Naloxiphan, RO-1-7700)

mg/kg		Mouse	Rat	Guinea Pig	Rabbit	Cat	Dog	Monkey	
Lethal Dose Y—LD$_{50}$ Z—MLD	IV								
	IP	Y184 [210]	Y185 [210]						
	IM								
	SC								
	PO		Y949 [210]						
Morphine Antagonist	IV				0.45 [1011]		0.2		
	IP								
	IM								
	SC	0.3 [908]							
	PO								
EEG (Desynchroni-zation)	IV				10 [157]	10 [184]			
	IP								
	IM								
	SC								
	PO								
Cardiovascular and Respiratory	IV				10 [157]				
	IP								
	IM								
	SC		125 [908]						
	PO								
Behavioral	IV								
	IP	6 [989]							
	IM								
	SC								
	PO								
Analgetic	IV								
	IP								
	IM								
	SC	2.4 [908]							
	PO								

LIDOCAINE

(Lignocaine, Xylocaine, Xylotox)

mg/kg		Mouse	Rat	Guinea Pig	Rabbit	Cat	Dog	Monkey	
Lethal Dose Y−LD$_{50}$ Z−MLD	IV	Y31.5 [436]							
	IP								
	IM								
	SC	Y400 [437]							
	PO	Y457 [1012]							
Anticonvulsant	IV					2.5 [440]		3 [442]	
	IP	75 [925]							
	IM								
	SC	4.9 [252]							
	PO	13 [1012]			25 [1012]				
Convulsant	IV				10 [438]	20 [440]			
	IP			>60 [991]					
	IM								
	SC								
	PO								
EEG and ECP	IV				5 [439]	16 [1214]			
	IP								
	IM								
	SC								
	PO				30 [1012]				
Block Afferent Nerve Discharge	IV						20 [441]		
	IP								
	IM								
	SC								
	PO								
Cardiovascular	IV						3 [1234]		
	IP								
	IM								
	SC								
	PO								

LIDOCAINE (continued)

mg/kg		Mouse	Rat	Guinea Pig	Rabbit	Cat	Dog	Monkey	
	IV								
	IP								
	IM								
	SC								
	PO								
	IV								
	IP								
	IM								
	SC								
	PO								
	IV								
	IP								
	IM								
	SC								
	PO								
	IV								
	IP								
	IM								
	SC								
	PO								

IN VITRO

mg %	Cardiac	Vascular	Gut	Uterine	Visceral	Skeletal		
Rat						5 [1157]		
Guinea Pig			0.3 [1157]					
	1 [1228]							

LYSERGIDE

(Delysid, LSD-25)

mg/kg		Mouse	Rat	Guinea Pig	Rabbit	Cat	Dog	Monkey	
Lethal Dose $Y-LD_{50}$ $Z-MLD$	IV	Y54 [443]			2 [92]				
	IP								
	IM								
	SC								
	PO								
Behavioral	IV				0.5 [446]	0.4	0.5 [446]	0.01 [452]	
	IP	4 [369]	2 [833]	10 [833]		0.02 [447]		0.1 [185]	
	IM	1 [175]				0.1 [448]		0.025 [289]	
	SC	2.5 [940]							
	PO	5 [935]							
Hyperthermic	IV				0.05 [443]				
	IP		4 [444]						
	IM								
	SC				0.06				
	PO								
EEG and ECP	IV				0.04	0.1 [184]	0.1 [451]		
	IP		2 [833]	10 [833]			0.04 [1196]		
	IM								
	SC								
	PO								
Pentobarbital Antagonist	IV				0.14 [159]				
	IP					50 [449]			
	IM								
	SC								
	PO								
Metabolic	IV					0.3 [450]			
	IP		1.3 [1239]						
	IM								
	SC		0.625 [445]						
	PO								

LYSERGIDE (continued)

mg/kg		Mouse	Rat	Guinea Pig	Rabbit	Cat	Dog	Monkey	
Antiseroton-ergic	IV		0.025 [386]			0.05 [453]			
	IP								
	IM								
	SC	0.03 [1014]		0.013 [917]					
	PO		1 [997]						
Ataxic	IV								
	IP								
	IM							0.1 [161]	
	SC								
	PO								
Catatonic	IV								
	IP								
	IM							1.0 [161]	
	SC								
	PO								
Fetal Damage	IV								
	IP								
	IM								
	SC		0.005 [1094]						
	PO		0.02 [1094]						

IN VITRO

mg %	Cardiac	Vascular	Gut	Uterine	Visceral	Skeletal		
Antiserotonergic				0.002 [443]				

MAGNESIUM SULFATE

(Epsom Salts)

mg/kg		Mouse	Rat	Guinea Pig	Rabbit	Cat	Dog	Monkey	
Lethal Dose Y−LD$_{50}$ Z−MLD	IV	1100 [97]	1100 [97]	1100 [97]	1100 [97]	1100 [97]	750	1100 [97]	
	IP						1600 [109]		
	IM								
	SC			Z1800 [454]	Z1750 [454]	Z1000 [454]	1750 [109]		
	PO								
CNS Depressant	IV								
	IP								
	IM								
	SC								
	PO				1.3				
DFP Antagonist	IV								
	IP								
	IM				400				
	SC								
	PO								
	IV								
	IP								
	IM								
	SC								
	PO								

IN VITRO

mg %	Cardiac	Vascular	Gut	Uterine	Visceral	Skeletal		

MEBUTAMATE

(Capla)

mg/kg		Mouse	Rat	Guinea Pig	Rabbit	Cat	Dog	Monkey	
Lethal Dose Y−LD$_{50}$ Z−MLD	IV								
	IP	Y460 [457]	Y410 [457]						
	IM								
	SC								
	PO	Y550 [457]	Y1160 [457]						
Cardiovascular	IV					30 [467]	20 [457]		
	IP				18 [457]				
	IM								
	SC								
	PO		120 [457]						
Anticonvulsant	IV								
	IP	90 [457]							
	IM								
	SC								
	PO								
	IV								
	IP								
	IM								
	SC								
	PO								

IN VITRO

mg %	Cardiac	Vascular	Gut	Uterine	Visceral	Skeletal		

mg/kg		Mouse	Rat	Guinea Pig	Rabbit	Cat	Dog	Monkey	
Lethal Dose $Y-LD_{50}$ $Z-MLD$ (as base)	IV	Y21 [58]							
	IP	Y39 [58]	Y54 [58]	Y52 [58]					
	IM								
	SC	Y93 [58]	Y145 [58]	Y127 [58]					
	PO	Y92 [58]	Y171 [58]	Y144 [58]			50 [58]		
Ganglionic Block (as base)	IV	2.5 [58]	2 [386]			0.23 [113]	1 [58]		
	IP	2.5 [58]							
	IM								
	SC								
	PO	2.5 [58]					2 [58]		
Cardiovascular	IV				10 [1133]	0.15 [867]	1 [458]		
	IP								
	IM								
	SC								
	PO								
Neuromuscular Block	IV						10 [214]		
	IP								
	IM								
	SC								
	PO								
Behavioral	IV								
	IP	2.5 [878]							
	IM								
	SC								
	PO	5 [935]							
Decreased Renshaw Cell Activity	IV					2.5 [1015]			
	IP								
	IM								
	SC								
	PO								

MEPENZOLATE

(Cantil)

mg/kg		Mouse	Rat	Guinea Pig	Rabbit	Cat	Dog	Monkey	
Lethal Dose $Y-LD_{50}$ $Z-MLD$	IV	Y9.8 460	Y21.8 460						
	IP								
	IM								
	SC								
	PO	Y900 460	Y1100 460						
Anticholinergic	IV					0.02 460	0.02 460		
	IP		5 460		0.015 460				
	IM								
	SC								
	PO								
	IV								
	IP								
	IM								
	SC								
	PO								
	IV								
	IP								
	IM								
	SC								
	PO								

IN VITRO

mg %	Cardiac	Vascular	Gut	Uterine	Visceral	Skeletal		
Anticholinergic			0.2 460					
Antihistaminic			200 460					

MEPHENESIN
(Myanesin, Tolseram, Tolseron)

mg/kg		Mouse	Rat	Guinea Pig	Rabbit	Cat	Dog	Monkey	
Lethal Dose Y–LD$_{50}$ Z–MLD	IV	Y186 909			Y125 845				
	IP	Y471 461	283 461						
	IM								
	SC	600 1221							
	PO	Y990 461	Y625 975						
Skeletal Muscle Relaxant (Central)	IV	30.9 909			35 845	20 845		100 1073	
	IP	400 204	120						
	IM								
	SC	180 1221					200		
	PO	550 462							
Strychnine Antagonist	IV								
	IP	100							
	IM		80						
	SC	200							
	PO	225 1016							
Polysynaptic Reflex Inhibition	IV		7 1142			20 1080	25 271		
	IP								
	IM								
	SC								
	PO								
Righting Reflex Loss	IV						150	125 1073	
	IP	130 461	103 461						
	IM								
	SC								
	PO	462 461	580 461						
Behavioral	IV								
	IP								
	IM								
	SC								
	PO	400 935	430 975						

149

MEPHENTERMINE

(Mephine, Vialin, Wyamine)

mg/kg		Mouse	Rat	Guinea Pig	Rabbit	Cat	Dog	Monkey	
Lethal Dose	IV								
$Y-LD_{50}$	IP	Y110 [464]							
$Z-MLD$	IM								
	SC								
	PO								
Cardiovascular	IV					1 [465]	4 [466]		
	IP								
	IM								
	SC								
	PO								
Increased Coronary Blood Flow	IV						1 [467]		
	IP								
	IM								
	SC								
	PO								
	IV								
	IP								
	IM								
	SC								
	PO								

IN VITRO

mg %	Cardiac	Vascular	Gut	Uterine	Visceral	Skeletal		
Adrenolytic	0.1 [468]		1.0 [465]					

mg/kg		Mouse	Rat	Guinea Pig	Rabbit	Cat	Dog	Monkey	
Lethal Dose $Y-LD_{50}$ $Z-MLD$	IV								
	IP		270 475	Y215 352					
	IM								
	SC								
	PO	Y560 352			Y430 352	Y190 352			
Ataxic	IV								
	IP								
	IM								
	SC								
	PO	103 352			33 352	6.3 352			
Behavioral	IV								
	IP	64 1155							
	IM								
	SC								
	PO								
	IV								
	IP								
	IM								
	SC								
	PO								

IN VITRO

mg %	Cardiac	Vascular	Gut	Uterine	Visceral	Skeletal		

MEPROBAMATE

(Equanil, Miltown, Quaname)

mg/kg		Mouse	Rat	Guinea Pig	Rabbit	Cat	Dog	Monkey	
Lethal Dose Y−LD$_{50}$ Z−MLD	IV	450 [211]	Y350		Y260 [845]				
	IP	Y710 [461]	410 [461]						
	IM								
	SC	550 [17]							
	PO	Y980 [461]	918 [461]						
Behavioral	IV					30 [254]			
	IP	100 [469]	135 [470]			20 [145]			
	IM	100 [175]						150 [1017]	
	SC	50 [1008]	300 [231]					400 [211]	
	PO	200 [924]	115 [211]		20 [417]	50 [211]	100 [417]	100 [211]	
Sedative	IV	200 [211]				45 [462]			
	IP	200 [211]	300 [463]			400 [1018]			
	IM								
	SC	180 [211]							
	PO	100	150 [117]	100 [472]		65 [557]	30 [557]	325 [473]	
Spinal Cord Depressant	IV					40 [1080]			
	IP								
	IM								
	SC								
	PO	185 [1016]							
Cardiovascular	IV				25 [471]		20 [839]		
	IP								
	IM								
	SC								
	PO								
Hypnotic	IV	270 [211]							
	IP	260 [211]							
	IM								
	SC	300 [211]							
	PO	348 [211]	659 [471]	300 [1019]					

mg/kg		Mouse	Rat	Guinea Pig	Rabbit	Cat	Dog	Monkey	
Anticonvulsant	IV								
	IP	155 461			100 474	20 110			
	IM								
	SC								
	PO	200 474	20 982	20 982					
Barbiturate Sleep Potentiation	IV								
	IP	80 469							
	IM								
	SC				100 142				
	PO		200 200	100 142					
Paralytic	IV	200 211			110 1171	20 1171			
	IP	200 211	300 463						
	IM								
	SC	180 211							
	PO	302 119	382 119						
EEG	IV				110 845	30 823			
	IP		40 1069						
	IM								
	SC								
	PO					160 1165			

IN VITRO

mg %	Cardiac	Vascular	Gut	Uterine	Visceral	Skeletal		

MESCALINE

(Mezcaline)

mg/kg		Mouse	Rat	Guinea Pig	Rabbit	Cat	Dog	Monkey	
Lethal Dose Y−LD$_{50}$ Z−MLD	IV								
	IP	Y500 115							
	IM								
	SC								
	PO	*Y1180 960							
CNS	IV				1.1 159		20 478		
	IP								
	IM								
	SC	30 119				50 476			
	PO								
Cardiovascular Respiratory	IV				25 157	7.5 477	5 478		
	IP								
	IM								
	SC								
	PO								
Behavioral	IV					1 110			
	IP		5 921						
	IM	50 251					70 479		
	SC								
	PO								
Decreased Spontaneous Motor Activity	IV								
	IP	50 813							
	IM								
	SC								
	PO	100 960							
EEG	IV					20 842			
	IP								
	IM								
	SC								
	PO								

*Caged individually.

METARAMINOL

(Aramine, Pressonex)

mg/kg		Mouse	Rat	Guinea Pig	Rabbit	Cat	Dog	Monkey	
Lethal Dose	IV	Y51 [58]							
Y—LD$_{50}$	IP		Y41						
Z—MLD	IM								
(as base)	SC	Y92 [58]	Y117 [58]						
	PO	Y99 [58]	Y240						
Cardiovascular	IV						0.07 [58]		
(as base)	IP								
	IM								
	SC		3 [862]						
	PO								
Catechol Amine Depletion	IV						0.25 [58]		
	IP	0.1 [58]		0.2 [58]					
(Heart)	IM								
	SC								
	PO								
	IV								
	IP								
	IM								
	SC								
	PO								

IN VITRO

mg %	Cardiac	Vascular	Gut	Uterine	Visceral	Skeletal		

METHACHOLINE

(Acetyl-β-methylcholine, Mecholyl)

mg/kg		Mouse	Rat	Guinea Pig	Rabbit	Cat	Dog	Monkey	
Lethal Dose $Y-LD_{50}$ $Z-MLD$	IV	Y15 [14]	Y20 [14]						
	IP								
	IM								
	SC	Y90 [14]	Y75 [14]						
	PO	Y1100 [14]	Y750 [14]						
Cholinergic	IV				0.002 [14]		0.002	7 [4]	
	IP					0.15 [4]		10 [4]	
	IM				5	0.15 [4]		10 [4]	
	SC				0.2 [14]	0.15 [4]		10 [4]	
	PO				50 [14]				
Cathartic	IV								
	IP								
	IM								
	SC						0.05 [14]		
	PO						25 [14]		
	IV								
	IP								
	IM								
	SC								
	PO								

IN VITRO

mg %	Cardiac	Vascular	Gut	Uterine	Visceral	Skeletal		
Rat				0.02 [1157]				
Rabbit	0.008 [1157]							

156

METHADONE

(Dolophine, Polamidon, Physeptone)

mg/kg		Mouse	Rat	Guinea Pig	Rabbit	Cat	Dog	Monkey	
Lethal Dose $Y-LD_{50}$ $Z-MLD$	IV	Y17 480	Y10 481				26		
	IP	Y38 480	Y23 480						
	IM								
	SC	Y33 480	Y12 480	Y54 480			52	Y15 480	
	PO	Y93.7 480	Y95						
Analgetic	IV								
	IP	5	20						
	IM								
	SC	20	13 482	10			4		
	PO						1.1 24		
Cardiovascular Respiratory	IV				3 43		5		
	IP								
	IM								
	SC								
	PO								
Behavioral	IV					10 1022			
	IP	2.5 251	10 483						
	IM								
	SC	1 1021	4.5 927						
	PO								
Eyelid Retraction (Central Sympathetic)	IV								
	IP								
	IM								
	SC	1 1086							
	PO								
	IV								
	IP								
	IM								
	SC								
	PO								

METHAMPHETAMINE

(Desoxyn, Methedrine, Pervitin)

mg/kg		Mouse	Rat	Guinea Pig	Rabbit	Cat	Dog	Monkey	
Lethal Dose Y−LD$_{50}$ Z−MLD	IV	Y10 111							
	IP	Y15 111	25 485						
	IM								
	SC	180				50			
	PO	*Y232 960	4 335						
Increased Motor Activity	IV	0.5 149	1 149						
	IP	2 149	2 149						
	IM	1 175							
	SC	5 484	0.3 200			2 149			
	PO	2 149	2 149			2 149			
Behavioral	IV								
	IP	20 177	0.5 1095			5 487			
	IM								
	SC		3.2 486						
	PO		10 973			2 1007	1 149		
Analgetic	IV							0.5 248	
	IP								
	IM								
	SC								
	PO								
Analeptic	IV				2 111				
	IP								
	IM								
	SC								
	PO								
Diuretic	IV								
	IP								
	IM								
	SC						4 885		
	PO								

*Caged individually.

mg/kg		Mouse	Rat	Guinea Pig	Rabbit	Cat	Dog	Monkey	
Lethal Dose Y—LD$_{50}$ Z—MLD	IV								
	IP	Y500 [111]							
	IM								
	SC								
	PO	Y500 [111]							
Anticonvulsant	IV				20 [111]				
	IP								
	IM								
	SC								
	PO	25 [111]			50 [111]		50 [111]		
Ataxic	IV								
	IP	150 [111]							
	IM								
	SC								
	PO	200 [111]							
	IV								
	IP								
	IM								
	SC								
	PO								

IN VITRO

mg %	Cardiac	Vascular	Gut	Uterine	Visceral	Skeletal		

METHOXAMINE

(Pressomin, Vasoxyl, Vasylox)

mg/kg		Mouse	Rat	Guinea Pig	Rabbit	Cat	Dog	Monkey	
Lethal Dose	IV	15 [149]							
Y−LD$_{50}$	IP	Y92 [488]							
Z−MLD	IM								
	SC								
	PO	135 [149]							
Cardiovascular	IV					0.2 [489]	0.1 [490]		
	IP								
	IM						3 [149]		
	SC						0.8 [149]		
	PO						35 [149]		
Barbiturate Sleep Potentiation	IV								
	IP								
	IM								
	SC	8 [98]							
	PO								
Antiarrhythmic	IV								
	IP	35 [856]							
	IM								
	SC								
	PO								

IN VITRO

mg %	Cardiac	Vascular	Gut	Uterine	Visceral	Skeletal		
Guinea Pig	0.5 [149]			*0.05 [149]				
Rabbit			*0.05 [149]	*0.05 [149]				

*mM

METHSCOPOLAMINE

(Pamine, Mescopil, Proscomide)

mg/kg		Mouse	Rat	Guinea Pig	Rabbit	Cat	Dog	Monkey	
Lethal Dose Y−LD$_{50}$ Z−MLD	IV								
	IP								
	IM								
	SC								
	PO								
Anticholinergic (Antisecretory)	IV		0.002 [491]						
	IP								
	IM				0.025 [491]		0.01 [491]		
	SC	1 [1087]	0.2 [491]						
	PO		14 [491]				1.5 [491]		
Neuromuscular Block	IV						25 [491]		
	IP								
	IM								
	SC								
	PO								
Ganglionic Block	IV					5 [491]			
	IP								
	IM								
	SC								
	PO								
CNS (Stimulant)	IV								
	IP								
	IM								
	SC		5 [491]						
	PO		50 [491]						
	IV								
	IP								
	IM								
	SC								
	PO								

α-METHYLDOPA

(Aldomet)

mg/kg		Mouse	Rat	Guinea Pig	Rabbit	Cat	Dog	Monkey	
Lethal Dose Y—LD$_{50}$ Z—MLD	IV	Y1900 [58]							
	IP	Y406 [58]	Y647 [58]						
	IM								
	SC								
	PO	Y5300 [58]	Y7490 [58]		Y713 [58]				
Decarboxylase Inhibition	IV		20 [493]	100 [494]		100 [493]			
	IP								
	IM								
	SC	100 [492]							
	PO								
Decreased Serotonin (Brain)	IV								
	IP								
	IM								
	SC	400 [492]		400 [492]					
	PO								
Catechol Amine Depletion (Heart)	IV	50 [58]					100 [58]		
	IP		400 [1141]						
	IM								
	SC								
	PO								
Barbiturate Sleep Potentiation	IV								
	IP								
	IM								
	SC	100 [492]							
	PO								
Cardiovascular	IV								
	IP		50 [1243]						
	IM								
	SC		213.8 [916]						
	PO		200 [1138]						

mg/kg		Mouse	Rat	Guinea Pig	Rabbit	Cat	Dog	Monkey	
Lethal Dose $Y-LD_{50}$ $Z-MLD$	IV	Y85 352	Y23 352		Y2.6 352				
	IP								
	IM								
	SC								
	PO	Y187 352	Y93 352						
Oxytocic	IV				0.2 352	0.125 352			
	IP								
	IM								
	SC								
	PO								
	IV								
	IP								
	IM								
	SC								
	PO								
	IV								
	IP								
	IM								
	SC								
	PO								

IN VITRO

mg %	Cardiac	Vascular	Gut	Uterine	Visceral	Skeletal		

METHYLPHENIDATE

(Phenidylate, Ritalin)

mg/kg		Mouse	Rat	Guinea Pig	Rabbit	Cat	Dog	Monkey	
Lethal Dose	IV	41 1025	Y48 115						
Y−LD50	IP	Y450 174							
Z−MLD	IM								
	SC	*Y470 1142							
	PO	*Y680 960	Y367 115						
CNS (Stimulant)	IV				5 495		2 93		
	IP	30 174							
	IM								
	SC	10 93	3.19 85					10 89	
	PO	50 960					10 93		
Antagonize Amphetamine Hypertension	IV					10 497	20 497		
	IP								
	IM								
	SC								
	PO								
Phentolamine Antagonist	IV						15 498		
	IP								
	IM								
	SC								
	PO								
Cardiovascular	IV		5 157		5 495	5 496	5 496		
	IP								
	IM								
	SC								
	PO								
Behavioral	IV								
	IP	10 1131							
	IM								
	SC	10 940	10 1026			2 1024			
	PO	80 935				2 1007			

*Caged individually.

164

mg/kg		Mouse	Rat	Guinea Pig	Rabbit	Cat	Dog	Monkey	
Lethal Dose $Y-LD_{50}$ $Z-MLD$	IV	275 307	Y237 481						
	IP	Y500	920 500		Y500 500				
	IM			Z400 502					
	SC	Y531 499	Y572 501	Y391 480	Y600 109	Z60	210 109		
	PO	Y745 911	Y905 481	Z1000 502					
Analgetic Preanesthetic	IV		20 503		2 1031		4	0.5 248	
	IP	2.3 309	5	12.1 22	5				
	IM		10	2-5 1221	2-5 1221		2-5 1221	0.5 248	
	SC	7.0 267	1.6 267	5 923	10 978		4		
	PO	52.5 267	15.4 267	25 978					
Behavioral	IV					1 1027			
	IP	10 1029	10.25 505			2 926			
	IM								
	SC	50 504	1.3 506	25 978		1 507	5 479		
	PO	25.4 701	40 1030						
Cardiovascular	IV		0.33 507		0.56 1133	1	4		
	IP								
	IM								
	SC		1.1 908		2 508		10 1028		
	PO								
Catatonic	IV							20 506	
	IP	100 1156							
	IM								
	SC	40	125				10 1028		
	PO		500 269						
EEG and ECP	IV		50 989		2 337	3 509	20 509		
	IP		10 1213						
	IM								
	SC					0.3 1205			
	PO								

mg/kg		Mouse	Rat	Guinea Pig	Rabbit	Cat	Dog	Monkey	
Convulsant	IV								
	IP								
	IM								
	SC		160 [1135]		500	20			
	PO								
Polysynaptic Reflex Inhibition	IV					0.4 [828]	1 [849]		
	IP								
	IM								
	SC		4 [1030]						
	PO								
Antibradykinin	IV								
	IP								
	IM								
	SC		1.1 [908]						
	PO								
Metabolic	IV								
	IP		50 [1209]						
	IM								
	SC		5 [1227]						
	PO								

IN VITRO

mg %	Cardiac	Vascular	Gut	Uterine	Visceral	Skeletal		
Rabbit	1		5					

mg/kg		Mouse	Rat	Guinea Pig	Rabbit	Cat	Dog	Monkey	
Lethal Dose Y−LD$_{50}$ Z−MLD	IV	Y0.23 [16]							
	IP								
	IM								
	SC				30 [511]	2.8 [109]			
	PO	750			268 [511]	28.6 [109]			
Spasmogenic	IV			0.002 [16]	0.01 [16]	0.005 [16]	0.0005 [16]		
	IP								
	IM								
	SC								
	PO								
Cardiovascular	IV			0.005 [16]	0.005 [16]	0.001 [16]	0.0005 [16]		
	IP								
	IM								
	SC								
	PO								
EEG (activation)	IV				1.2 [1100]	0.0001 [826]			
	IP								
	IM								
	SC								
	PO								

IN VITRO

mg %	Cardiac	Vascular	Gut	Uterine	Visceral	Skeletal		
Guinea Pig	0.002 [16]		0.002 [16]	0.01 [16]	0.002 [16]			
Rabbit	0.003 [16]		0.003 [16]	0.05 [16]	0.008 [16]			
Dog			0.0008 [16]	0.01 [16]	0.0003 [16]			

NALORPHINE

(Allorphine, Lethidrone, Nalline)

mg/kg		Mouse	Rat	Guinea Pig	Rabbit	Cat	Dog	Monkey	
Lethal Dose	IV	Y190 [58]							
$Y - LD_{50}$	IP	Y590 [17]						.	
$Z - MLD$	IM								
	SC	Y670 [58]							
	PO								
Morphine Antagonist (10 times Morphine Dose)	IV				5 [513]	3 [514]	2		
	IP	5 [512]	5			0.2 [1032]			
	IM						0.4 [97]		
	SC	5 [1033]	2 [58]				15		
	PO								
Analgetic	IV					8 [891]			
	IP	13.8 [17]	1.55 [513]						
	IM								
	SC	100 [515]							
	PO								
EEG	IV				0.004 [516]	8 [891]			
	IP								
	IM								
	SC								
	PO								
Antidepressant	IV								
	IP								
	IM								
	SC			10 [90]					
	PO								
Decreased Polysynaptic Reflex	IV						1 [849]		
	IP					.			
	IM								
	SC								
	PO								

mg/kg		Mouse	Rat	Guinea Pig	Rabbit	Cat	Dog	Monkey	
Lethal Dose $Y-LD_{50}$ $Z-MLD$	IV	Y0.36 [517]	Y0.16 [518]		0.25 [519]		20 [521]		
	IP	Y0.62 [907]							
	IM				Y0.31 [517]				
	SC	Y0.8 [517]	Y0.37 [518]		Z12.5 [520]		Z13.5 [520]		
	PO	Y14.4 [517]							
Cholinergic	IV					0.1 [1034]	0.025		
	IP								
	IM					1 [1034]			
	SC						0.025		
	PO								
Anticurare	IV		0.1 [1143]		0.25	0.025	0.17		
	IP								
	IM								
	SC		0.3						
	PO								
Anticonvulsant	IV								
	IP								
	IM								
	SC	1 [957]							
	PO								

IN VITRO

mg %	Cardiac	Vascular	Gut	Uterine	Visceral	Skeletal		
Rabbit		0.25	0.25					
Rat						0.01 [1157]		

NIALAMIDE

(Niamid, P-1133)

mg/kg		Mouse	Rat	Guinea Pig	Rabbit	Cat	Dog	Monkey	
Lethal Dose $Y-LD_{50}$ $Z-MLD$	IV								
	IP	Y742 [115]							
	IM								
	SC								
	PO	Y1000 [115]	Y1700 [115]						
Monoamine-oxidase Inhibition (Brain)	IV				100 [522]				
	IP		*0.25 [1169]	*10 [1169]					
	IM							25 [1170]	
	SC		30 [173]			10 [173]			
	PO								
Behavioral	IV								
	IP			150 [1036]					
	IM								
	SC		100 [1010]			10 [173]			
	PO								
Anticonvulsant	IV								
	IP	100 [523]	35 [1035]						
	IM								
	SC								
	PO								
EEG (Synchronization)	IV								
	IP								
	IM								
	SC					10 [173]			
	PO								
CNS Stimulant	IV					50 [861]			
	IP								
	IM								
	SC								
	PO								

*for 6 days

mg/kg		Mouse	Rat	Guinea Pig	Rabbit	Cat	Dog	Monkey	
Lethal Dose Y–LD$_{50}$ Z–MLD	IV	Y7.1 [524]	Z1	Z4.5 [527]	Y9.4 [524]		Y5 [524]		
	IP	10							
	IM								
	SC	Z16 [525]	Y33.5 [526]	Z27.5 [528]	20 [528]				
	PO	Z24 [525]	Y55						
Behavioral	IV	0.3 [529]	0.23 [530]		0.02 [533]	0.02 [533]			
	IP	5 [369]	5.0 [531]						
	IM				0.2 [967]	0.05 [1151]			
	SC	0.4 [1101]	0.5 [532]				0.2 [534]		
	PO	10 [935]							
Cardiovascular	IV			0.3	0.1 [535]	0.2 [101]	0.25		
	IP								
	IM								
	SC						0.1		
	PO								
EEG	IV		1 [1150]	1.5 [1150]	0.01 [825]	0.01 [825]	0.01 [825]	0.01 [825]	
	IP								
	IM								
	SC				0.2 [1203]				
	PO								
Gastrointestinal	IV					0.05 [1093]			
	IP								
	IM								
	SC		0.15 [1242]						
	PO								
Increased Spinal Cord Inhibition	IV					0.3 [1037]			
	IP								
	IM								
	SC								
	PO								

NICOTINE (continued)

mg/kg		Mouse	Rat	Guinea Pig	Rabbit	Cat	Dog	Monkey	
	IV								
	IP								
	IM								
	SC								
	PO								
	IV								
	IP								
	IM								
	SC								
	PO								
	IV								
	IP								
	IM								
	SC								
	PO								
	IV								
	IP								
	IM								
	SC								
	PO								

IN VITRO

mg %	Cardiac	Vascular	Gut	Uterine	Visceral	Skeletal		
Rabbit	0.1		0.25					
Guinea Pig			0.2 [1157]					
Rat			0.5 [1157]					
Spasmogenic			0.5 [1233]					

NIKETHAMIDE

(Anacardone, Coramine, Tonocard)

mg/kg		Mouse	Rat	Guinea Pig	Rabbit	Cat	Dog	Monkey	
Lethal Dose Y−LD$_{50}$ Z−MLD	IV		Y191 [93]		250 [5]		175 [537]		
	IP	Y174 [284]	Y300 [537]	250 [537]	Y225 [537]				
	IM						175 [537]		
	SC	295 [536]	Y470 [538]	300 [537]	350 [537]				
	PO				650 [537]				
Analeptic	IV	19 [1137]			10		75		
	IP								
	IM						75		
	SC						75		
	PO								
Behavioral CNS	IV				45 [157]		33 [24]		
	IP								
	IM	100 [175]							
	SC			50 [978]			33 [24]		
	PO								
Convulsant	IV								
	IP	145 [284]							
	IM								
	SC	201 [284]							
	PO								
Antiserotonergic	IV			10 [92]					
	IP								
	IM								
	SC								
	PO								
	IV								
	IP								
	IM								
	SC								
	PO								

NITROGLYCEROL

(Glyceryl Trinitrate, Perglottal, Trinitroglycerol)

mg/kg		Mouse	Rat	Guinea Pig	Rabbit	Cat	Dog	Monkey	
Lethal Dose Y—LD$_{50}$ Z—MLD	IV				Z45 [346]				
	IP								
	IM		Z275 [346]		Z450 [346]				
	SC				500 [346]	200 [346]			
	PO		Z100						
Cardiovascular (anesthetized)	IV						0.05		
	IP								
	IM								
	SC						0.01		
	PO		20 [539]						
Cardiovascular (conscious)	IV						0.025 [1218]		
	IP								
	IM								
	SC								
	PO								
	IV								
	IP								
	IM								
	SC								
	PO								

IN VITRO

mg %	Cardiac	Vascular	Gut	Uterine	Visceral	Skeletal		

mg/kg		Mouse	Rat	Guinea Pig	Rabbit	Cat	Dog	Monkey	
Lethal Dose Y$-$LD$_{50}$ Z$-$MLD	IV								
	IP								
	IM								
	SC								
	PO								
Cardiovascular	IV					0.3 $_{912}$	0.3 $_{912}$		
	IP								
	IM								
	SC								
	PO								
	IV								
	IP								
	IM								
	SC								
	PO								
	IV								
	IP								
	IM								
	SC								
	PO								

IN VITRO

mg %	Cardiac	Vascular	Gut	Uterine	Visceral	Skeletal		

OUABAIN

(Astrobain, Gratibain, G-Strophanthin)

mg/kg		Mouse	Rat	Guinea Pig	Rabbit	Cat	Dog	Monkey	
Lethal Dose Y−LD$_{50}$ Z−MLD	IV		17.2 [540]		0.2 [303]	Y0.11	0.12 [542]		
	IP	Y20							
	IM			Y0.26 [541]					
	SC	10 [303]	Y97 [166]	0.2 [303]	0.25 [303]	0.17 [303]	0.13 [303]		
	PO				14 [303]	2.4 [109]	1.5 [109]		
Cardiac	IV			0.02	0.05	0.089 [913]	0.025		
	IP								
	IM						0.025 [97]		
	SC								
	PO								
Arrhythmic	IV				0.05 [1090]		0.05		
	IP								
	IM								
	SC								
	PO								
Emetic	IV					0.06 [890]	0.05 [1013]		
	IP								
	IM								
	SC								
	PO								

IN VITRO

mg %	Cardiac	Vascular	Gut	Uterine	Visceral	Skeletal		
Rabbit	0.063		0.05					

mg/kg		Mouse	Rat	Guinea Pig	Rabbit	Cat	Dog	Monkey	
Lethal Dose $Y-LD_{50}$ $Z-MLD$	IV	Y33.1 [543]							
	IP	Y750	Y63 [546]						
	IM								
	SC	Z500 [544]	Y420 [1128]		Z250 [109]				
	PO	Y2500 [545]	Y745 [543]						
Cardiovascular	IV			10			7		
	IP			50 [1219]					
	IM								
	SC								
	PO								
Catatonic	IV								
	IP								
	IM								
	SC					30 [476]			
	PO								
Behavioral	IV								
	IP	60 [1131]							
	IM								
	SC								
	PO								

IN VITRO

mg %	Cardiac	Vascular	Gut	Uterine	Visceral	Skeletal		
Guinea Pig			0.001					
Rabbit	5		7.5					
Antiserotonergic			0.3 [92]					

PARACHLOROPHENYLALANINE

(PCPA)

mg/kg		Mouse	Rat	Guinea Pig	Rabbit	Cat	Dog	Monkey	
Lethal Dose Y−LD$_{50}$ Z−MLD	IV								
	IP								
	IM								
	SC								
	PO								
Hypersexuality	IV								
	IP		*100 $_{1184}$		*100 $_{1186}$				
	IM								
	SC								
	PO								
Deplete Brain Serotonin and Histamine	IV								
	IP		310 $_{1188}$						
	IM								
	SC								
	PO								
Behavioral	IV								
	IP		320 $_{1190}$						
	IM								
	SC								
	PO								

*daily, 3-5 days

IN VITRO

mg %	Cardiac	Vascular	Gut	Uterine	Visceral	Skeletal		

mg/kg		Mouse	Rat	Guinea Pig	Rabbit	Cat	Dog	Monkey	
Lethal Dose Y–LD$_{50}$ Z–MLD	IV				Y450 [7]	Y450 [7]	Y500 [7]		
	IP	Z1500 [547]		Y1230 [549]					
	IM								
	SC	Z1650 [547]							
	PO	Y1650 [548]			5000 [109]		Y3500 [109]		
Anesthetic	IV				300 [7]	300 [7]	300 [7]		
	IP								
	IM								
	SC								
	PO				1000		2000		
Anticonvulsant	IV								
	IP	500 [1038]							
	IM								
	SC	266 [1075]							
	PO	1000 [550]							
Behavioral (Ataxic)	IV								
	IP								
	IM								
	SC	462 [1075]							
	PO	800 [935]							

IN VITRO

mg %	Cardiac	Vascular	Gut	Uterine	Visceral	Skeletal		

PARGYLINE

(A-19120, Eutonyl, MO-911)

mg/kg		Mouse	Rat	Guinea Pig	Rabbit	Cat	Dog	Monkey	
Lethal Dose $Y-LD_{50}$ $Z-MLD$	IV								
	IP	Y370 [551]	Y142 [551]			Y200 [551]		Y150 [551]	
	IM								
	SC								
	PO	Y680 [551]	Y300 [551]				Y175 [551]		
Monoamine-oxidase Inhibition	IV		10 [1215]		10 [552]				
	IP	10 [69]	20 [1118]						
	IM		25 [867]						
	SC		12 [868]						
	PO	75 [69]							
Increased Tissue Norepinephrine	IV				25 [552]				
	IP	100 [551]	50 [553]		100 [830]	100 [553]			
	IM								
	SC								
	PO								
Reverse Reserpine Depression (with DOPA)	IV				50 [69]		25 [1130]		
	IP								
	IM								
	SC								
	PO							50 [551]	
Behavioral (irritability)	IV								
	IP								
	IM								
	SC								
	PO						100 [554]		
CNS	IV					30 [861]			
	IP								
	IM								
	SC								
	PO								

PENTOBARBITAL
(Embutal, Mebubarbital, Nembutal)

mg/kg		Mouse	Rat	Guinea Pig	Rabbit	Cat	Dog	Monkey	
Lethal Dose Y−LD$_{50}$ Z−MLD	IV	Y80 555	Z50		Y45 394		62 111		
	IP	Y130 555	Y75	Y50 556	Z65 129	Z60 449	Z50		
	IM	Y124 555		Y70 1235					
	SC	Y107 1075	125 66						
	PO	Y280 555	Y118		Y275 394	Y100 558			
Anesthetic	IV	35 111	25 111	30 111	30 111	25 111	30 111	25 111	
	IP	60 111	*50 111	35 111	40 111	38 111	38 111	30 111	
	IM		50 902	20 1235		15 557			
	SC						30 111		
	PO	80 111	50 111	50 111	45 111	50 111	50 111	45 111	
Behavioral	IV				5 562	3.4 563		12 564	
	IP	27.8 903	10 470					15 185	
	IM							20 289	
	SC		20 231				8 895	20 977	
	PO	35 561	5 232			15 1108		20 929	
EEG and ECP	IV				10 559	5	10 560	5 945	
	IP		5 1069						
	IM								
	SC								
	PO						40 560		
Cardiovascular	IV					6 565	10 560		
	IP								
	IM								
	SC								
	PO								
Neuronal Membrane Stabilization	IV					10 566			
	IP								
	IM								
	SC								
	PO								

*see 1121 for sex differences

PENTOBARBITAL (continued)

mg/kg		Mouse	Rat	Guinea Pig	Rabbit	Cat	Dog	Monkey	
Ataxic	IV	12.9 ₅₆₆			15 ₅₆₂				
	IP								
	IM								
	SC	30 ₁₀₇₅	5 ₅₆₇						
	PO					15 ₁₁₀₈			
Tremor	IV								
	IP					30 ₅₆₈			
	IM								
	SC								
	PO								
Increased Serotonin (Brain)	IV								
	IP		50 ₃₁						
	IM								
	SC								
	PO								
Muscle Contraction (Denervated)	IV							25	
	IP								
	IM								
	SC								
	PO								
Anticonvulsant	IV								
	IP	26 ₁₁₁₅							
	IM								
	SC								
	PO								
Increased Brain Acetylcholine	IV								
	IP		50 ₁₂₀₉						
	IM								
	SC								
	PO								

mg/kg		Mouse	Rat	Guinea Pig	Rabbit	Cat	Dog	Monkey	
Lethal Dose Y−LD$_{50}$ Z−MLD	IV	Y29 [214]							
	IP	Y36 [214]							
	IM								
	SC								
	PO	Y512 [214]							
Ganglionic Block	IV					0.07 [113]	0.5		
	IP		5 [381]						
	IM								
	SC								
	PO								
Epinephrine Sensitization	IV					0.24 [154]			
	IP								
	IM								
	SC								
	PO								
Neuromuscular Block	IV						10 [214]		
	IP								
	IM								
	SC								
	PO								
Cardiovascular	IV				10 [1133]				
	IP								
	IM								
	SC								
	PO								
	IV								
	IP								
	IM								
	SC								
	PO								

PENTYLENETETRAZOL

(Cardiazol, Leptazol, Metrazol)

mg/kg		Mouse	Rat	Guinea Pig	Rabbit	Cat	Dog	Monkey	
Lethal Dose $Y-LD_{50}$ $Z-MLD$	IV	Y51 [962]	50 [569]		Z70 [572]	80 [570]	40		
	IP	Y92 [569]	Y70 [962]	90 [570]					
	IM								
	SC	Y101 [962]	Y100 [571]	85 [570]	87.5 [570]	75 [570]			
	PO	Y162 [962]	140 [962]						
Convulsant	IV	48 [121]	20 [573]		20	11	20 [134]		
	IP	40.5 [284]	64 [121]	47.5 [961]			60 [962]		
	IM	40 [251]	100			50 [918]		64 [575]	
	SC	85							
	PO	68 [284]	175 [574]						
Analeptic	IV				60		20		
	IP	10 [961]	57.5 [571]	40 [961]					
	IM						10		
	SC	19 [284]					10		
	PO								
Cardiovascular	IV				15 [157]		50 [410]		
	IP								
	IM								
	SC								
	PO								
Behavioral	IV								
	IP		20 [1145]			20 [1068]			
	IM	50 [175]							
	SC								
	PO	50 [935]							
EEG	IV				100 [974]	10 [1039]			
	IP								
	IM								
	SC								
	PO								

mg/kg		Mouse	Rat	Guinea Pig	Rabbit	Cat	Dog	Monkey	
Lethal Dose Y–LD$_{50}$ Z–MLD	IV	37 228	38 228			35 417	51 228		
	IP	Y70 1131	124 228						
	IM								
	SC								
	PO	120 228	318 228				100 228		
"Tranquilize"	IV				1.2 844				
	IP	3.8 1119							
	IM						0.5 228	0.2 576	
	SC	0.1 223	0.1 223			0.1 223	0.1 223	0.1 223	
	PO	1.0 223	1.0 223			1.0 223	1.0 223	1.5 223	
Behavioral	IV								
	IP	1 986	0.25 577			4 417			
	IM								
	SC	0.75 1040	0.4 578				0.4 1040	0.15 1041	
	PO	10 417	2 417			10 417	10 417		
Preanesthetic Medication	IV					0.55 97	0.55 97		
	IP								
	IM					0.55 97	0.55 97		
	SC								
	PO		10 417			0.88 97	0.88 97		
Adrenolytic	IV					1 417	1 417		
	IP								
	IM								
	SC								
	PO								
Cardiovascular	IV				1 471	2 417	2 417		
	IP								
	IM								
	SC								
	PO								

185

PERPHENAZINE (continued)

mg/kg		Mouse	Rat	Guinea Pig	Rabbit	Cat	Dog	Monkey	
EEG	IV				3 [417]				
	IP								
	IM								
	SC								
	PO								
Experimental Shock Protection	IV						1 [228]		
	IP								
	IM		1.5 [228]						
	SC								
	PO								
Ataxic	IV						2 [417]		
	IP								
	IM								
	SC		10 [1042]						
	PO								
Decerebrate Rigidity Abolished	IV					0.4 [844]			
	IP								
	IM								
	SC								
	PO								

IN VITRO

mg %	Cardiac	Vascular	Gut	Uterine	Visceral	Skeletal		

mg/kg		Mouse	Rat	Guinea Pig	Rabbit	Cat	Dog	Monkey	
Lethal Dose Y−LD$_{50}$ Z−MLD	IV	Y50 579	Y34 580		Y30 579		100		
	IP	Y150	Y93 580						
	IM								
	SC	Y195 579	Y200 579						
	PO	Y178 579	Y170		Y500 579				
Analgetic Sedative	IV	20 1043	10 269			10 191	2		
	IP	40	50 580	51.8 22					
	IM			2 1235		7.5	10		
	SC	60	43.6 581	20.4 1044		11 1232	25		
	PO	46.9 1126	150 580			11 24	11 24		
Spinal Reflex Depressant	IV					13 510			
	IP								
	IM								
	SC		100 269						
	PO								
Cardiovascular	IV						2 860		
	IP								
	IM								
	SC								
	PO								

IN VITRO

mg %	Cardiac	Vascular	Gut	Uterine	Visceral	Skeletal		
Rabbit	20		20					

PHENACEMIDE

(Carbanmide, Phenurone, Epiclase)

mg/kg		Mouse	Rat	Guinea Pig	Rabbit	Cat	Dog	Monkey	
Lethal Dose Y—LD$_{50}$ Z—MLD	IV								
	IP								
	IM								
	SC								
	PO	Y5000 [111]			3500 [111]	2000 [111]	3500 [111]		
Anticonvulsant	IV								
	IP	80 [933]							
	IM								
	SC								
	PO	300 [111]	21 [851]		300 [111]		*1100 [97]		
Behavioral	IV								
	IP								
	IM								
	SC								
	PO	205							
Ataxic	IV								
	IP								
	IM								
	SC								
	PO	400 [111]							
	IV								
	IP								
	IM								
	SC								
	PO								
	IV								
	IP								
	IM								
	SC								
	PO								

*Total dose

PHENAZONE

(Analgesine, Anti-Pyrine, Pyrazolin)

mg/kg		Mouse	Rat	Guinea Pig	Rabbit	Cat	Dog	Monkey	
Lethal Dose Y—LD$_{50}$ Z—MLD	IV				700 [109]				
	IP	Z1000 [4]							
	IM	Z1000 [4]							
	SC	1000 [109]		1000 [109]	1250 [109]	700 [109]			
	PO	Y1800 [109]	Y1800 [18]	1400 [109]			750 [109]		
Analgetic Antipyretic	IV								
	IP	197 [1045]			100 [4]	100 [4]			
	IM				100 [4]	100 [4]			
	SC		600 [21]		100 [4]	100 [4]			
	PO		220 [18]		500 [4]	500 [4]	*1000 [97]		
Anti-inflammatory	IV								
	IP								
	IM								
	SC								
	PO			100 [55]					
	IV								
	IP								
	IM								
	SC								
	PO								

*Total dose

IN VITRO

mg %	Cardiac	Vascular	Gut	Uterine	Visceral	Skeletal		

PHENCYCLIDINE

mg/kg		Mouse	Rat	Guinea Pig	Rabbit	Cat	Dog	Monkey	
Lethal Dose Y−LD$_{50}$ Z−MLD	IV								
	IP								
	IM								
	SC								
	PO								
Anesthetic	IV					1.1 1232		1 1073	
	IP								
	IM							1.5 1073	
	SC								
	PO								
Behavioral	IV							0.3 1073	
	IP	5 1073							
	IM								
	SC								
	PO								
Convulsant	IV							4 1073	
	IP	50 1073							
	IM								
	SC								
	PO								

IN VITRO

mg %	Cardiac	Vascular	Gut	Uterine	Visceral	Skeletal		

PHENELZINE

(Alazine, Nardelzine, Nardil)

mg/kg		Mouse	Rat	Guinea Pig	Rabbit	Cat	Dog	Monkey	
Lethal Dose $Y-LD_{50}$ $Z-MLD$	IV	Y157 [115]							
	IP								
	IM								
	SC	Y150 [1046]							
	PO	Y156 [115]	210 [455]						
Analgetic	IV								
	IP								
	IM								
	SC								
	PO	12 [582]							
Respiratory	IV								
	IP	10 [455]							
	IM								
	SC								
	PO	15 [455]							
Monoamine Oxidase Inhibition	IV	48 [608]							
	IP	32 [608]	10 [1118]						
	IM								
	SC		10 [1046]						
	PO		10 [1046]						
Cardiovascular	IV					0.6 [608]	5 [583]		
	IP					15 [608]			
	IM								
	SC								
	PO								
Behavioral	IV								
	IP		5 [848]						
	IM								
	SC								
	PO								

PHENIPRAZINE

(Catron, JB-516, Catroniazid)

mg/kg		Mouse	Rat	Guinea Pig	Rabbit	Cat	Dog	Monkey	
Lethal Dose $Y-LD_{50}$ $Z-MLD$	IV	Y60.6 [460]	Y44.5 [460]			35 [584]			
	IP	Y122	50						
	IM								
	SC	Y95 [460]	Y45.3 [460]			35 [584]			
	PO	Y73 [460]	Y34.1 [460]						
Monoamine-oxidase Inhibition	IV	3 [430]			3 [430]	1.5	5 [372]		
	IP		20 [584]				15		
	IM		10 [867]						
	SC	3 [430]			2 [430]	1.5 [91]			
	PO								
CNS Behavioral	IV				5 [584]	25 [584]	10 [586]		
	IP	50 [585]	30 [585]				25 [584]		
	IM								
	SC		20 [460]		2 [430]	25 [584]			
	PO								
Cardiovascular	IV		10 [218]	5	5	5	5 [372]		
	IP								
	IM								
	SC								
	PO								
Barbiturate Sleep Potentiation	IV								
	IP	10 [585]	10 [585]						
	IM								
	SC								
	PO								
	IV								
	IP								
	IM								
	SC								
	PO								

PHENOBARBITAL

(Gardenal, Luminal, Sental)

mg/kg		Mouse	Rat	Guinea Pig	Rabbit	Cat	Dog	Monkey	
Lethal Dose Y−LD$_{50}$ Z−MLD	IV				Y185 122	100 1232			
	IP	Y340 122	Y190 122		Z150 588	150 1232			
	IM				Z150 128				
	SC	Y230	Y200 68						
	PO	Y325 391	Y660 587		Z150 588	Y175 558			
Anesthetic	IV	134 65	100 589		200 590	*60 97	80 591		
	IP			100		180	150	100	
	IM					*60 97	30 557		
	SC	96					30 557		
	PO	107		30 76		*60 97	150	125	
Anticonvulsant	IV				25 594	20 846	25 594		
	IP	25 592	25 592					15 595	
	IM							15 1096	
	SC	20	30 414		50				
	PO	25	25 593	70 1047		*45 24	*150 24		
Behavioral	IV						1 947		
	IP	100 933	15 470			40 1147		27 1230	
	IM	40 175	30 230						
	SC		39 596						
	PO	90 505	80 934	4 1047		40 1165	75 597		
Cardiovascular	IV				50 598		20 599		
	IP								
	IM								
	SC								
	PO								
Ataxic	IV								
	IP								
	IM								
	SC	69 1075	88 596						
	PO	250 484				40 1165			

*Total dose

PHENOBARBITAL (continued)

mg/kg		Mouse	Rat	Guinea Pig	Rabbit	Cat	Dog	Monkey	
Antidiuretic	IV						40 [591]		
	IP								
	IM								
	SC				120 [591]				
	PO								
Reflex Depressant	IV					10 [564]			
	IP								
	IM								
	SC								
	PO								
EEG	IV				40 [1223]	40 [843]			
	IP					20 [1009]			
	IM								
	SC								
	PO				40 [1012]				
	IV								
	IP								
	IM								
	SC								
	PO								

IN VITRO

mg %	Cardiac	Vascular	Gut	Uterine	Visceral	Skeletal		

PHENOXYBENZAMINE

(Dibenzyline)

mg/kg		Mouse	Rat	Guinea Pig	Rabbit	Cat	Dog	Monkey	
Lethal Dose $Y-LD_{50}$ $Z-MLD$	IV						Z 10 [82]		
	IP								
	IM								
	SC								
	PO	Y 15 35 [82]	Y 2500 [82]	Y 500 [82]					
Adrenolytic (α-block)	IV	5 [1197]	0.031 [253]		15 [220]	3.0 [404]	15		
	IP		1 [383]						
	IM								
	SC								
	PO								
CNS	IV				1.5 [87]	0.6 [873]			
	IP	5 [350]	1 [1243]			10 [1100]			
	IM								
	SC		5 [350]						
	PO								
Catecholamine Depletion	IV					10 [901]	20 [816]		
	IP		10 [600]						
	IM								
	SC								
	PO								
Decreased Blood Pressure	IV				1 [1133]	5 [1085]			
	IP		0.2 [387]	100 [1219]					
	IM								
	SC								
	PO		50 [387]						
EEG (Synchronization)	IV				1.5 [298]				
	IP								
	IM								
	SC								
	PO								

PHENOXYBENZAMINE (continued)

mg/kg		Mouse	Rat	Guinea Pig	Rabbit	Cat	Dog	Monkey	
Shock (therapy)	IV						0.1		
	IP								
	IM								
	SC								
	PO								
Block Amphetamine Hyperthermia	IV				5 [1182]				
	IP								
	IM								
	SC								
	PO								
	IV								
	IP								
	IM								
	SC								
	PO								
	IV								
	IP								
	IM								
	SC								
	PO								

IN VITRO

mg %	Cardiac	Vascular	Gut	Uterine	Visceral	Skeletal		
Adrenolytic		0.005		0.005	0.006			
Spasmolitic			0.1 [1223]					

PHENTOLAMINE

(C-7337, Regitine, Rogitine)

mg/kg		Mouse	Rat	Guinea Pig	Rabbit	Cat	Dog	Monkey	
Lethal Dose Y-LD_{50} Z-MLD	IV		Y75 603						
	IP								
	IM								
	SC		Y275 603						
	PO	Y1000 119	Y1250 603						
Adrenolytic (α-block)	IV		10 218		3 305	2 497	1 408		
	IP	4 939		10 1219					
	IM								
	SC				1 603	1 603	1 603		
	PO						20 1082		
CNS	IV				0.25 914				
	IP								
	IM								
	SC								
	PO	150 119							
Cardiac	IV					0.5 821			
	IP								
	IM								
	SC								
	PO								
Anticonvulsant	IV								
	IP								
	IM								
	SC	10 957							
	PO								
Bronchiol Dilation	IV								
	IP								
	IM								
	SC			4.5 1081					
	PO								

PHENTOLAMINE (continued)

mg/kg		Mouse	Rat	Guinea Pig	Rabbit	Cat	Dog	Monkey	
Increase Norepinephrine from Spleen	IV					3 [901]			
	IP								
	IM								
	SC								
	PO								
	IV								
	IP								
	IM								
	SC								
	PO								
	IV								
	IP								
	IM								
	SC								
	PO								
	IV								
	IP								
	IM								
	SC								
	PO								

IN VITRO

mg %	Cardiac	Vascular	Gut	Uterine	Visceral	Skeletal		
Adrenolytic		0.008 [1157]	0.01 [604]					
Antiserotonergic			0.1 [92]					
Rabbit			0.04 [1157]					

198

mg/kg		Mouse	Rat	Guinea Pig	Rabbit	Cat	Dog	Monkey	
Lethal Dose $Y-LD_{50}$ $Z-MLD$	IV	Y123 [605]							
	IP	Y336 [17]	Y215 [605]						
	IM								
	SC								
	PO	Y1150 [923]	Y650 [923]						
Analgetic	IV				100 [50]				
	IP	150 [50]							
	IM								
	SC	5.6 [908]							
	PO	200 [923]		300 [923]					
Anti-inflammatory	IV								
	IP		100 [928]						
	IM								
	SC		200 [50]						
	PO		90 [326]	1800 [55]					
Antipyretic	IV								
	IP								
	IM								
	SC				20 [905]				
	PO	200 [935]	12.5 [905]						
Antibradykinin	IV								
	IP		32 [908]						
	IM								
	SC								
	PO								
	IV								
	IP								
	IM								
	SC								
	PO								

PHENYLEPHRINE

(Adrianol, Meta-Sympatol, Neosynephrine)

mg/kg		Mouse	Rat	Guinea Pig	Rabbit	Cat	Dog	Monkey	
Lethal Dose $Y-LD_{50}$ $Z-MLD$	IV	Y21 840	6.8 607						
	IP	Y1000					16 840		
	IM								
	SC	Y70 840	Y92 1128						
	PO	Y120 840	Y350 1128						
Cardiovascular	IV			0.04		0.01 840	0.03 408		
	IP	2 840							
	IM								
	SC								
	PO	50 840							
CNS (Stimulant)	IV								
	IP								
	IM								
	SC						0.5		
	PO								
	IV								
	IP								
	IM								
	SC								
	PO								

IN VITRO

mg %	Cardiac	Vascular	Gut	Uterine	Visceral	Skeletal		
Rabbit	0.04		0.01					

PHENYTOIN

(Dilantin, Diphenylhydantoin, Eptoin)

mg/kg		Mouse	Rat	Guinea Pig	Rabbit	Cat	Dog	Monkey	
Lethal Dose $Y - LD_{50}$ $Z - MLD$	IV		Z160 610		Y125 70		Z90 610		
	IP	Y200 609	Y280 70						
	IM								
	SC								
	PO	Y490 226	Z > 2200 610						
Anticonvulsant	IV					30 613			
	IP	20 611	135 612		60				
	IM							15 1097	
	SC	75	300		55				
	PO	50	2200 610		35 1012		*50 24		
Toxic Dose (Emesis)	IV						5		
	IP	800	200		40 1068				
	IM								
	SC								
	PO	84 226							
Tremorine Antagonist	IV								
	IP								
	IM	99 140							
	SC								
	PO	60 1131							
Behavioral	IV							40 1048	
	IP		50 1145						
	IM		50 230			†15 1229			
	SC								
	PO								
Cardiovascular	IV				30 818	2-20 1211	5 818		
	IP								
	IM								
	SC								
	PO								

*Total dose

†on 2 successive days

PHENYTOIN (continued)

mg/kg		Mouse	Rat	Guinea Pig	Rabbit	Cat	Dog	Monkey	
Vagus Nerve Depression	IV						20 [818]		
	IP								
	IM								
	SC								
	PO								
Respiratory Depression	IV				30 [818]		20 [818]		
	IP								
	IM								
	SC								
	PO								
Uterin Activity Depression	IV				40 [819]		20 [819]		
	IP								
	IM								
	SC								
	PO								
EEG	IV				40 [1223]	20 [1222]			
	IP								
	IM								
	SC								
	PO								

IN VITRO

mg %	Cardiac	Vascular	Gut	Uterine	Visceral	Skeletal		
Rabbit				0.1 [819]				

mg/kg		Mouse	Rat	Guinea Pig	Rabbit	Cat	Dog	Monkey	
Lethal Dose $Y-LD_{50}$ $Z-MLD$	IV	0.5 [519]			0.4 [614]	0.25 [614]			
	IP	Y1 [907]							
	IM								
	SC	Y1.12 [907]			3 [519]				
	PO	Y3.0 [115]							
Cholinergic	IV						0.5		
	IP								
	IM								
	SC				1 [88]	0.5 [944]	1		
	PO								
EEG (desynchroni- zation)	IV				0.3 [60]	0.1 [1034]			
	IP								
	IM								
	SC								
	PO								
Behavioral	IV					0.3 [1034]	0.1	0.3 [871]	
	IP	0.5 [852]	0.8 [1144]			0.2 [1100]			
	IM								
	SC	0.3 [856]	1 [1049]			10 [944]			
	PO	1 [935]							
Increased Spinal Cord Inhibition	IV					1.5 [379]			
	IP								
	IM								
	SC								
	PO								
Bulbocapnine Potentiation	IV				0.1 [288]				
	IP	0.05 [615]							
	IM								
	SC								
	PO								

203

PHYSOSTIGMINE (continued)

mg/kg		Mouse	Rat	Guinea Pig	Rabbit	Cat	Dog	Monkey	
Tremor	IV								
	IP	5 [369]	0.75 [1118]						
	IM								
	SC								
	PO								
Hypothermic	IV								
	IP	0.5 [1087]							
	IM								
	SC								
	PO								
	IV								
	IP								
	IM								
	SC								
	PO								
	IV								
	IP								
	IM								
	SC								
	PO								

IN VITRO

mg %	Cardiac	Vascular	Gut	Uterine	Visceral	Skeletal		
Rabbit	0.025		0.5					
Rat						0.01 [1157]		
Guinea Pig	0.08 [1157]							

PICROTOXIN

(Cocculin)

mg/kg		Mouse	Rat	Guinea Pig	Rabbit	Cat	Dog	Monkey	
Lethal Dose Y−LD$_{50}$ Z−MLD	IV	Z4	Y3 166		Z1.25 617				
	IP	Y7.2 284	Y6.5 166						
	IM								
	SC	Y7.04 284	4.7 616	8 109	Z2.5 617		2.2 109		
	PO	Y14.8 284							
Analeptic	IV			12.6 1235	3		0.3		
	IP	10 123				1.5 618	0.3		
	IM						0.3		
	SC	1.6 284					0.3		
	PO								
CNS (Stimulant)	IV	2.9 121	2.9 121		0.89 121	0.2 854	*2 24		
	IP		9 130			0.5 1068			
	IM								
	SC	5.9 121	3 617						
	PO								
Convulsant	IV					0.3 134			
	IP	4.8 284							
	IM								
	SC	3.14 284			3 869				
	PO	8.43 284							
Behavioral	IV								
	IP								
	IM	1 175							
	SC		0.5 1050						
	PO								
Cardiovascular	IV						2 886		
	IP								
	IM								
	SC								
	PO								

*Total dose

PILOCARPINE

mg/kg		Mouse	Rat	Guinea Pig	Rabbit	Cat	Dog	Monkey	
Lethal Dose Y$-$LD$_{50}$ Z$-$MLD	IV				175 [109]				
	IP	Y500							
	IM								
	SC								
	PO								
Cholinergic	IV						3		
	IP								
	IM					*2 [24]	*12 [24]		
	SC		160 [619]		5	*2 [24]	0.75		
	PO								
Anticonvulsant	IV								
	IP								
	IM								
	SC	160 [620]	26 [620]						
	PO								
Spinal Cord Inhibition Blocked	IV					80 [900]			
	IP								
	IM								
	SC								
	PO								
Hypothermic	IV								
	IP	10 [1087]	5 [1111]						
	IM								
	SC								
	PO								
EEG (arousal)	IV				0.64 [1099]				
	IP								
	IM								
	SC								
	PO								

*Total dose

mg/kg		Mouse	Rat	Guinea Pig	Rabbit	Cat	Dog	Monkey	
Lethal Dose Y−LD$_{50}$ Z−MLD	IV								
	IP								
	IM								
	SC								
	PO								
	IV								
	IP								
	IM								
	SC								
	PO								
	IV								
	IP								
	IM								
	SC								
	PO								
	IV								
	IP								
	IM								
	SC								
	PO								

IN VITRO

mg %	Cardiac	Vascular	Gut	Uterine	Visceral	Skeletal		
Rabbit	0.5		1	1				

PIPRADROL

(Meratran, MRD-108, Piridol)

mg/kg		Mouse	Rat	Guinea Pig	Rabbit	Cat	Dog	Monkey	
Lethal Dose $Y-LD_{50}$ $Z-MLD$	IV		Y30 115		Y15 117				
	IP	Y94 115							
	IM								
	SC	Y240 115	Y240 117						
	PO	*Y365 960	Y180 115						
CNS Stimulant and Increased Motor Activity	IV		6 117						
	IP	10 323							
	IM								
	SC	20 204	2.74 85						
	PO	50 960							
Analeptic	IV				12.5 117		2 133		
	IP		20 621						
	IM								
	SC								
	PO								
Cardiovascular	IV					8 117			
	IP								
	IM								
	SC								
	PO								
Behavioral	IV								
	IP		5 622						
	IM								
	SC						1 1051		
	PO								
	IV								
	IP								
	IM								
	SC								
	PO								

*Caged individually.

mg/kg		Mouse	Rat	Guinea Pig	Rabbit	Cat	Dog	Monkey	
Lethal Dose $Y-LD_{50}$ $Z-MLD$	IV	2.5 [109]	Z2.5 [195]				5		
	IP	Z6 [109]							
	IM		8						
	SC	Y6.02 [273]	Z17 [195]						
	PO	Y16 [623]	Z12.5 [195]		Y5		1.6 [624]		
Vagal Bradycardia Potentiation	IV					0.03 [625]			
	IP								
	IM								
	SC								
	PO								
Increased O_2 Consumption	IV								
	IP								
	IM								
	SC		9.6 [626]						
	PO								
	IV								
	IP								
	IM								
	SC								
	PO								

IN VITRO

mg %	Cardiac	Vascular	Gut	Uterine	Visceral	Skeletal		

PROBARBITAL

(Ipral)

mg/kg		Mouse	Rat	Guinea Pig	Rabbit	Cat	Dog	Monkey	
Lethal Dose	IV				140 27				
Y−LD$_{50}$	IP	250 66	110 66		110 66				
Z−MLD	IM								
	SC		310 66						
	PO				160 66	140 66			
Anesthetic	IV								
	IP	75 66			66 66				
	IM								
	SC		225 66						
	PO								
	IV								
	IP								
	IM								
	SC								
	PO								
	IV								
	IP								
	IM								
	SC								
	PO								

IN VITRO

mg %	Cardiac	Vascular	Gut	Uterine	Visceral	Skeletal		

PROBENECID

(Benemid)

mg/kg		Mouse	Rat	Guinea Pig	Rabbit	Cat	Dog	Monkey	
Lethal Dose Y−LD$_{50}$ Z−MLD	IV	Y458 [627]			Y304 [627]		Y270 [627]		
	IP		Y394 [627]						
	IM								
	SC	Y1156 [627]	Y611 [627]						
	PO	Y1666 [627]	Y1604 [627]						
Uricosuric	IV						16 [58]		
	IP								
	IM								
	SC								
	PO		300 [58]				30 [58]		
	IV								
	IP								
	IM								
	SC								
	PO								
	IV								
	IP								
	IM								
	SC								
	PO								

IN VITRO

mg %	Cardiac	Vascular	Gut	Uterine	Visceral	Skeletal		

PROCAINE

(Allocaine, Neocaine, Novocaine)

mg/kg		Mouse	Rat	Guinea Pig	Rabbit	Cat	Dog	Monkey	
Lethal Dose Y−LD$_{50}$ Z−MLD	IV	Y45 [111]	Y50	Y51 [629]	Y57 [249]	Z45	Y62.4 [7]		
	IP	Y230 [111]	Y250 [166]	Z60					
	IM	Y630 [628]	Y1600 [111]						
	SC	Y800 [259]	Y2100 [259]	Z430	Z460	Z450	Z250		
	PO	Y500 [111]							
Convulsant	IV				30				
	IP								
	IM			100 [630]					
	SC						100		
	PO								
Block Afferent Nerve Discharge	IV					10 [292]	20 [441]		
	IP								
	IM								
	SC								
	PO								
Decreased Intestinal Motility and Pain	IV					10 [440]			
	IP								
	IM								
	SC								
	PO								
Cardiovascular	IV				20 [631]	20 [631]	20 [631]		
	IP								
	IM								
	SC								
	PO								
	IV								
	IP								
	IM								
	SC								
	PO								

PROCHLORPERAZINE

(Compazine, Novamin, Stemetil)

mg/kg		Mouse	Rat	Guinea Pig	Rabbit	Cat	Dog	Monkey	
Lethal Dose Y−LD$_{50}$ Z−MLD	IV	Y92 982	20 235		5 235		Z100 82		
	IP	Y125 982							
	IM								
	SC	Y350 982							
	PO	Y750 982	Y1800 82				Z102 82		
Behavioral	IV								
	IP		8 227						
	IM							0.1 1053	
	SC	10 561	1.3 95						
	PO	7.4 505	2.5 934						
Cardiovascular	IV					0.1 82	0.5 82		
	IP								
	IM								
	SC								
	PO		0.05 82						
Decreased Activity	IV								
	IP	10 986							
	IM								
	SC	1 578							
	PO								
Catatonic	IV				30 1052				
	IP	11.3 1052	16.5 227						
	IM								
	SC		30 1042						
	PO								
EEG (Synchroni- zation)	IV				2 824				
	IP								
	IM				5				
	SC								
	PO								

213

PROCHLORPERAZINE (continued)

mg/kg		Mouse	Rat	Guinea Pig	Rabbit	Cat	Dog	Monkey	
Hypothermic	IV								
	IP								
	IM								
	SC	8.5 [983]							
	PO								
	IV								
	IP								
	IM								
	SC								
	PO								
	IV								
	IP								
	IM								
	SC								
	PO								
	IV								
	IP								
	IM								
	SC								
	PO								

IN VITRO

mg %	Cardiac	Vascular	Gut	Uterine	Visceral	Skeletal		
Spasmolytic			0.1					
Anticholinergic			*0.8 [235]					
Antihistaminic		*0.11 [235]	*0.002 [235]					
Antiserotonergic			*0.0005 [235]					

*Total mg

214

mg/kg		Mouse	Rat	Guinea Pig	Rabbit	Cat	Dog	Monkey	
Lethal Dose $Y-LD_{50}$ $Z-MLD$	IV	Y91 [267]	Y74 [267]						
	IP								
	IM								
	SC	Y194 [267]	Y188 [267]						
	PO	Y318 [267]	Y253 [267]						
Analgetic	IV	30 [267]	11.2 [267]						
	IP								
	IM		26.3 [267]						
	SC	72.3 [267]	17.8 [267]						
	PO	84 [267]	17.3 [267]						
Emetic	IV								
	IP								
	IM						2.5 [267]		
	SC					60 [267]	10 [267]		
	PO					60 [267]	10 [267]		
Cardiovascular	IV					10 [267]	10 [267]		
	IP								
	IM								
	SC								
	PO								
Convulsant	IV								
	IP								
	IM								
	SC					80 [267]		60 [267]	
	PO								
	IV								
	IP								
	IM								
	SC								
	PO								

PROMAZINE

(Protactyl, Sparine, Verophene)

mg/kg		Mouse	Rat	Guinea Pig	Rabbit	Cat	Dog	Monkey	
Lethal Dose $Y-LD_{50}$ $Z-MLD$	IV	Y38 235	Y29 235		Y21 235				
	IP								
	IM						Y4.4 557		
	SC								
	PO	Y485 226	Y650 986						
Sedative and EEG (Synchronization)	IV				2 632	3.3 97	1.5		
	IP								
	IM					3.3 97	5.5 557		
	SC								
	PO	40 119				3.3 97	9 557		
Behavioral	IV								
	IP	5 633	2.4 227					7 1230	
	IM								
	SC	15 1054	3 986						
	PO	10 986	200 986						
Adrenolytic	IV		0.041 253						
	IP	10 634							
	IM								
	SC								
	PO								
Analgetic	IV								
	IP	10 238	120 238						
	IM								
	SC								
	PO	100 231							
Flexor Reflex Depression	IV								
	IP				1 238				
	IM								
	SC								
	PO								

mg/kg		Mouse	Rat	Guinea Pig	Rabbit	Cat	Dog	Monkey	
Barbiturate Sleep Potentiation	IV						2 425		
	IP	14.4 227							
	IM								
	SC	5 118				4.4 1232			
	PO		50 986						
Catatonic	IV								
	IP		3.3 227						
	IM								
	SC		25 1042						
	PO								
Anticonvulsant	IV								
	IP	5 982	5 982	5 982					
	IM								
	SC								
	PO								
Reverse Amphetamine EEG Arousal	IV				1 835				
	IP								
	IM								
	SC								
	PO								

IN VITRO

mg %	Cardiac	Vascular	Gut	Uterine	Visceral	Skeletal		
Anticholinergic			*0.175 235					
Antihistaminic		0.04 235	*0.004 235					
Antiserotonergic			*0.0006 235					
Anti-BaCl$_2$			*0.0002 235					

*Total mg

217

PROMETHAZINE

(Atosil, Phenergan, Thiergan)

mg/kg		Mouse	Rat	Guinea Pig	Rabbit	Cat	Dog	Monkey	
Lethal Dose Y—LD$_{50}$ Z—MLD	IV	Y75 235	Y45 235	Y42.5 629	Y19 235				
	IP								
	IM								
	SC	Y750	Y225						
	PO	Y125 88							
Anticonvulsant	IV								
	IP	40							
	IM								
	SC	72 252							
	PO								
Barbiturate Sleep Potentiation	IV								
	IP	12.5 1055							
	IM								
	SC	20 88	10 88				5 88		
	PO								
Sympatho- mimetic Sensitization	IV					15 635			
	IP	40 251							
	IM								
	SC								
	PO								

IN VITRO

mg %	Cardiac	Vascular	Gut	Uterine	Visceral	Skeletal		
Antihistaminic		0.006 235	0.01					
Anticholinergic			1 88					
Antiserotonergic			*0.0007 235					
Adrenolytic				0.1 88				

*Total mg

mg/kg		Mouse	Rat	Guinea Pig	Rabbit	Cat	Dog	Monkey	
Motion Sickness Antagonist	IV								
	IP		28.2 [1055]						
	IM						*125 [97]		
	SC								
	PO		312 [1056]						
EEG (synchronize)	IV				2 [824]	1 [1057]			
	IP								
	IM								
	SC								
	PO								
Behavioral	IV								
	IP	8 [1155]							
	IM								
	SC								
	PO								
	IV								
	IP								
	IM								
	SC								
	PO								

*Total dose

IN VITRO

mg %	Cardiac	Vascular	Gut	Uterine	Visceral	Skeletal		
Anti-BaCl$_2$			0.5 [88]					

PRONETHALOL

(Alderlin, Nethalide)

mg/kg		Mouse	Rat	Guinea Pig	Rabbit	Cat	Dog	Monkey	
Lethal Dose Y—LD_{50} Z—MLD	IV	Y50 636	Y50 636						
	IP	Y124 887							
	IM								
	SC								
	PO	Y900 636	Y900 636			300 636			
Adrenolytic (β-block)	IV		1.9 887			5 636	5 636		
	IP								
	IM								
	SC		20 1083						
	PO			6.8 887			10 636		
Decrease Norepinephrine Uptake (Heart)	IV								
	IP		2 919						
	IM								
	SC								
	PO								
CNS	IV								
	IP								
	IM								
	SC								
	PO					300 636	250 636		

IN VITRO

mg %	Cardiac	Vascular	Gut	Uterine	Visceral	Skeletal		
Adrenolytic	0.01		1 636					

mg/kg		Mouse	Rat	Guinea Pig	Rabbit	Cat	Dog	Monkey	
Lethal Dose $Y-LD_{50}$ $Z-MLD$	IV								
	IP								
	IM								
	SC								
	PO								
Adrenolytic (β-block)	IV	5 1197		2.5 1091	1 1112	3 1113	2 1088		
	IP	10 1153							
	IM								
	SC	10 1152			5 1120				
	PO								
Cardiovascular	IV		0.1 1127						
	IP		1 1243						
	IM								
	SC		0.5 1139						
	PO								
Antiarrythmic	IV				0.5 1090		10 1089		
	IP								
	IM								
	SC								
	PO						0.5 1194		
CNS (Behavioral)	IV						3 1154		
	IP								
	IM								
	SC								
	PO		10 877						
Metabolic	IV						4 1216		
	IP								
	IM								
	SC								
	PO								

PROPRANOLOL (continued)

mg/kg		Mouse	Rat	Guinea Pig	Rabbit	Cat	Dog	Monkey	
Block Ethanol Respiratory Depression	IV								
	IP	1 1237							
	IM								
	SC								
	PO								
	IV								
	IP								
	IM								
	SC								
	PO								
	IV								
	IP								
	IM								
	SC								
	PO								
	IV								
	IP								
	IM								
	SC								
	PO								

IN VITRO

mg %	Cardiac	Vascular	Gut	Uterine	Visceral	Skeletal		
Langendorff	*0.003 1157							
Rat				0.001 1157				
Rabbit	0.002 1157		3 1157					
	0.6 1228							

*Total mg.

222

mg/kg		Mouse	Rat	Guinea Pig	Rabbit	Cat	Dog	Monkey	
Lethal Dose Y−LD$_{50}$ Z−MLD	IV								
	IP								
	IM								
	SC		Y298 [1128]						
	PO		Y370 [1128]						
Anticholinergic	IV								
	IP		5 [144]						
	IM						5 [638]		
	SC		0.05 [637]						
	PO								
Ganglionic Block	IV					0.7 [113]			
	IP								
	IM								
	SC								
	PO								
Chromodac- ryorrhetic	IV								
	IP		0.29 [103]						
	IM								
	SC								
	PO								
	IV								
	IP								
	IM								
	SC								
	PO								
	IV								
	IP								
	IM								
	SC								
	PO								

PROTOVERATRINE

(Provell, Puroverine, Veralba)

mg/kg		Mouse	Rat	Guinea Pig	Rabbit	Cat	Dog	Monkey	
Lethal Dose Y−LD$_{50}$ Z−MLD	IV	Y0.05 [639]			Y0.05 [641]				
	IP	Y0.4 [640]							
	IM								
	SC		Y0.6 [639]		Y0.11 [639]	Y0.5 [641]			
	PO		Y5.0 [639]						
Cardiovascular	IV					0.002 [279]	0.001 [642]		
	IP								
	IM								
	SC		0.14 [916]						
	PO								
Respiratory (Depression)	IV						0.007 [643]		
	IP								
	IM								
	SC								
	PO								
	IV								
	IP								
	IM								
	SC								
	PO								

IN VITRO

mg %	Cardiac	Vascular	Gut	Uterine	Visceral	Skeletal		

PSEUDOEPHEDRINE

(Sudafed, d-ψ-Ephedrine, d-Isoephedrine)

mg/kg		Mouse	Rat	Guinea Pig	Rabbit	Cat	Dog	Monkey	
Lethal Dose Y—LD$_{50}$ Z—MLD	IV				85 [149]		125 [149]		
	IP								
	IM								
	SC		650 [149]		400 [149]				
	PO	115.5 [149]							
Cardiovascular	IV					1 [149]			
	IP								
	IM								
	SC								
	PO								
Diuretic	IV						0.6 [149]		
	IP								
	IM								
	SC								
	PO								
	IV								
	IP								
	IM								
	SC								
	PO								

IN VITRO

mg %	Cardiac	Vascular	Gut	Uterine	Visceral	Skeletal		
Contractile				0.3 [149]	0.2 [149]			

PSILOCIN

mg/kg		Mouse	Rat	Guinea Pig	Rabbit	Cat	Dog	Monkey	
Lethal Dose Y−LD$_{50}$ Z−MLD	IV	Y74 [115]	Y75 [115]						
	IP								
	IM								
	SC								
	PO								
Cardiovascular	IV						100 [158]		
	IP								
	IM								
	SC								
	PO								
EEG	IV				2 [906]				
	IP								
	IM								
	SC								
	PO								
	IV								
	IP								
	IM								
	SC								
	PO								

IN VITRO

mg %	Cardiac	Vascular	Gut	Uterine	Visceral	Skeletal		
Antiserotonergic			*0.0005 [644]	*0.00003 [644]				

*Total mg

mg/kg		Mouse	Rat	Guinea Pig	Rabbit	Cat	Dog	Monkey	
Lethal Dose Y−LD$_{50}$ Z−MLD	IV	Y285 [115]	Y280 [115]						
	IP								
	IM								
	SC								
	PO								
Behavioral	IV								
	IP		0.25 [921]						
	IM								
	SC								
	PO								
Cardiovascular	IV						0.2 [158]		
	IP		0.15 [155]						
	IM								
	SC								
	PO								
Pentobarbital EEG Antagonist	IV				0.32 [159]				
	IP								
	IM								
	SC								
	PO								

IN VITRO

mg %	Cardiac	Vascular	Gut	Uterine	Visceral	Skeletal		
Antiserotonergic			*0.006 [644]	0.001 [644]				

*Total mg

PSILOCYBIN (continued)

mg/kg		Mouse	Rat	Guinea Pig	Rabbit	Cat	Dog	Monkey	
Respiratory (Depression)	IV						0.5 645		
	IP								
	IM								
	SC								
	PO								
Increased Flexor Reflex	IV					0.2			
	IP								
	IM								
	SC								
	PO								
Decreased Catachoamines (Brain)	IV								
	IP		25 1239						
	IM								
	SC								
	PO								
	IV								
	IP								
	IM								
	SC								
	PO								

IN VITRO

mg %	Cardiac	Vascular	Gut	Uterine	Visceral	Skeletal		

PYRILAMINE

(Anthisan, Mepyramine, Neo-Antergan)

mg/kg		Mouse	Rat	Guinea Pig	Rabbit	Cat	Dog	Monkey	
Lethal Dose $Y-LD_{50}$ $Z-MLD$	IV	Y30 324		Y24.4 629					
	IP	Y102 646							
	IM								
	SC	Y150 324	Y150 647	Y70 324					
	PO	Y235 58							
Antihistaminic	IV			0.1 1122			5 649		
	IP								
	IM						75 97		
	SC			1.3 58			75 97		
	PO			11.3 648			*125 97		
Sympatho- mimetic (Sensitization)	IV					5 144			
	IP								
	IM								
	SC								
	PO								
Anticonvulsant	IV								
	IP		0.5 930						
	IM								
	SC								
	PO								

*Total dose

IN VITRO

mg %	Cardiac	Vascular	Gut	Uterine	Visceral	Skeletal		
Antihistaminic			0.003					
Guinea Pig			0.002 1157					

PYROCATECHOL

(Catechol, Pyrocatechin)

mg/kg		Mouse	Rat	Guinea Pig	Rabbit	Cat	Dog	Monkey	
Lethal Dose Y—LD$_{50}$ Z—MLD	IV						45 651		
	IP		100 1058	150 205					
	IM								
	SC	150 195	225 650	225 650					
	PO		Y3890		1000 346				
Cardiovascular	IV						100 652		
	IP		12 328						
	IM								
	SC								
	PO								
CNS (Stimulation)	IV					5 653			
	IP								
	IM								
	SC								
	PO								
EEG	IV				6 832				
	IP		50 1058						
	IM								
	SC								
	PO								

IN VITRO

mg %	Cardiac	Vascular	Gut	Uterine	Visceral	Skeletal		
Langendorff	*30 652							
Depressant	** 6 652							

*Total mg
**mmol/L

PYROGALLOL

(Pyrogallic Acid)

mg/kg		Mouse	Rat	Guinea Pig	Rabbit	Cat	Dog	Monkey	
Lethal Dose $Y-LD_{50}$ $Z-MLD$	IV						Z90 [651]		
	IP								
	IM								
	SC		Z650 [650]	Z1000 [650]			Z350 [654]		
	PO				Z1100 [109]		Z25 [346]		
Cardiovascular	IV		45			4 [655]	25 [282]		
	IP								
	IM								
	SC								
	PO								
Catechol-o-methyl Transferase Inhibition	IV					4 [655]			
	IP	*10 [656]	200 [811]						
	IM								
	SC								
	PO								
Chloral Hydrate Potentiation	IV								
	IP	50 [342]							
	IM								
	SC								
	PO								
	IV								
	IP								
	IM								
	SC								
	PO								
	IV								
	IP								
	IM								
	SC								
	PO								

*Total dose

QUINIDINE

(Quinicardine)

mg/kg		Mouse	Rat	Guinea Pig	Rabbit	Cat	Dog	Monkey	
Lethal Dose Y-LD$_{50}$ Z-MLD	IV	Y69 [555]	Y23.1 [363]			Y21.6 [658]			
	IP	Y190 [555]	Z174 [657]						
	IM	Y200							
	SC	Z400 [657]							
	PO	Y593.9 [555]	Y1000 [363]						
Block Atrial Flutter	IV			5		2 [659]	3		
	IP	72 [858]							
	IM								
	SC								
	PO								
Cardiovascular	IV				8.75 [1090]	10 [659]	15 [363]		
	IP								
	IM								
	SC								
	PO					15 [1134]	30 [1134]		
Nictitating Membrane Relaxation	IV					10 [363]	15 [363]		
	IP								
	IM								
	SC								
	PO								

IN VITRO

mg %	Cardiac	Vascular	Gut	Uterine	Visceral	Skeletal		
Guinea Pig				2				
Rabbit	5		1					

mg/kg		Mouse	Rat	Guinea Pig	Rabbit	Cat	Dog	Monkey	
Carotid Sinus Reflex Depressant	IV								
	IP								
	IM								
	SC								
	PO						30 [363]		
	IV								
	IP								
	IM								
	SC								
	PO								
	IV								
	IP								
	IM								
	SC								
	PO								
	IV								
	IP								
	IM								
	SC								
	PO								

IN VITRO

mg %		Cardiac	Vascular	Gut	Uterine	Visceral	Skeletal		

RESERPINE

(Sandril, Serpasil, Serpasol)

mg/kg		Mouse	Rat	Guinea Pig	Rabbit	Cat	Dog	Monkey	
Lethal Dose Y–LD$_{50}$ Z–MLD	IV		Y18 93				Y0.5 93		
	IP	Y70 1131							
	IM								
	SC								
	PO	Y500 176							
Sedative	IV		5 899		3.5 661	1 634	0.05		
	IP	2.5 79					0.05	5 161	
	IM	2 477							
	SC	2.5 93	5 660						
	PO	10 474	2 1221	4		10 634	0.65 93		
Serotonin and Norepinephrine Depletion	IV		0.4 662		5 667	3 91	5		
	IP	1 861	5 663	2.3 665		3 668	0.1 669		
	IM							1 1170	
	SC		5 664	0.1 666		5	5		
	PO								
Behavioral	IV		0.2 670		1 1023				
	IP	6 137	5 106		0.5 1068				
	IM		1 260			5 487		0.75 671	
	SC	2 561	1.2 596						
	PO	5 935	2 1059		2 1059	2 1059	2 1059		
CNS	IV				2 509	1 396			
	IP	0.5 882	0.5 1172			0.2 447			
	IM								
	SC								
	PO								
Barbituate Sleep Potentiation	IV		5 233				0.5 822		
	IP	5 469	5 411						
	IM								
	SC	1 1060							
	PO								

mg/kg		Mouse	Rat	Guinea Pig	Rabbit	Cat	Dog	Monkey	
Catatonic	IV								
	IP		5 165						
	IM								
	SC								
	PO								
Cardiovascular	IV		1.5 985	1	1 640	1 634	1 640		
	IP		2.5	10 1219	0.55 457				
	IM								
	SC		0.13 916						
	PO						1 640		
Metabolic	IV		1 884						
	IP								
	IM								
	SC								
	PO								
Anticonvulsant	IV								
	IP	4 1115							
	IM								
	SC	1 957							
	PO								

IN VITRO

mg %	Cardiac	Vascular	Gut	Uterine	Visceral	Skeletal		
Rabbit			0.1					
Antiserotonergic			3.0 92					

SCOPOLAMINE

(Hyoscine, Scopos)

mg/kg		Mouse	Rat	Guinea Pig	Rabbit	Cat	Dog	Monkey	
Lethal Dose Y–LD₅₀ Z–MLD	IV								
	IP								
	IM								
	SC	Y590 672							
	PO								
Anticholinergic	IV						0.06 915		
	IP	0.07 915	10 1118						
	IM								
	SC	5 673				0.5			
	PO		1.5 144						
Sedative	IV						1		
	IP								
	IM								
	SC	450 672	13 674				1		
	PO								
Increased Muscle Activity	IV								
	IP								
	IM								
	SC	20 176	5 491						
	PO		10 491						
EEG (Synchronization)	IV				0.08 675	0.1 184			
	IP								
	IM							1.5 945	
	SC		1.05 1173				1.5 945		
	PO								
Behavioral	IV				0.05 1161		0.32 915	0.1 1163	
	IP	1 852	1.8 106			0.6 1068		0.1 185	
	IM		0.6 1174						
	SC	1 856	1 1016				1.5 945		
	PO						1.5 945		

SCOPOLAMINE (continued)

mg/kg		Mouse	Rat	Guinea Pig	Rabbit	Cat	Dog	Monkey	
Anticonvulsant	IV								
	IP	5 [251]							
	IM								
	SC								
	PO								
Increased EEG Arousal Threshold	IV				0.1 [831]				
	IP								
	IM								
	SC								
	PO								
	IV								
	IP								
	IM								
	SC								
	PO								
	IV								
	IP								
	IM								
	SC								
	PO								

IN VITRO

mg %	Cardiac	Vascular	Gut	Uterine	Visceral	Skeletal		
Anticholinergic					*2.5×10^{-10}			
Antihistaminic					*7×10^{-5}			
Anti-BaCl$_2$					*1×10^{-4}			

* M/L

SECOBARBITAL

(Evronal, Seconal, Seotal)

mg/kg		Mouse	Rat	Guinea Pig	Rabbit	Cat	Dog	Monkey	
Lethal Dose Y−LD$_{50}$ Z−MLD	IV	Z80 [63]	Z35 [63]	Z35 [63]	Z45 [63]	Z50 [63]			
	IP	Z140 [63]	Z110 [63]	Z40 [63]	Z50 [63]	Z75 [63]			
	IM								
	SC	Z160 [63]	Z140 [63]	Z60 [63]	Z90 [63]				
	PO		Z125 [63]			Y50 [63]	Z90 [63]		
Anesthetic	IV	30 [63]	17.5 [63]	20 [63]	22.5 [72]	25 [63]		17.5 [63]	
	IP	60 [63]	40 [63]	20 [63]	30 [63]	35 [63]			
	IM								
	SC	70 [63]	60 [63]	30 [63]	50 [63]				
	PO		65 [63]	15 [76]			40 [63]		
Sedative	IV								
	IP		40 [63]						
	IM								
	SC		60 [63]						
	PO		65 [63]			3 [24]	3 [24]		
Serotonin Increase (Brain)	IV								
	IP		40						
	IM								
	SC								
	PO								
Flexor Reflex Inhibition	IV					5.4 [34]			
	IP								
	IM								
	SC								
	PO								
	IV								
	IP								
	IM								
	SC								
	PO								

mg/kg		Mouse	Rat	Guinea Pig	Rabbit	Cat	Dog	Monkey	
Lethal Dose	IV	Y125.6 550							
$Y-LD_{50}$	IP	Y123.3 550							
$Z-MLD$	IM								
	SC	Y125.5 550							
	PO	Y176 550							
Convulsant	IV	111.7 550					10 550		
	IP	116.4 550	150 550	75 550	175 550	40 550		60 550	
	IM								
	SC	250 1062							
	PO								
	IV								
	IP								
	IM								
	SC								
	PO								
	IV								
	IP								
	IM								
	SC								
	PO								

IN VITRO

mg %	Cardiac	Vascular	Gut	Uterine	Visceral	Skeletal		

SEROTONIN

(5-Hydroxytryptamine)

mg/kg		Mouse	Rat	Guinea Pig	Rabbit	Cat	Dog	Monkey	
Lethal Dose Y−LD_{50} Z−MLD	IV	Y160 [814]	Y30 [814]						
	IP	Y868 [814]	Y117 [814]						
	IM	Y750 [119]							
	SC								
	PO								
Cardiovascular Respiratory	IV		0.003		0.02 [158]	0.014 [676]	0.05 [282]		
	IP								
	IM								
	SC								
	PO								
Barbiturate Sleep Potentiation	IV		1.25 [677]						
	IP	8 [98]	10 [286]						
	IM								
	SC	50 [286]	50 [286]						
	PO								
EEG (Desynchroni-zation)	IV				0.065 [331]	0.05 [678]			
	IP								
	IM								
	SC								
	PO								
Anticonvulsant	IV								
	IP								
	IM								
	SC		50 [414]						
	PO								
Decreased Cold Exposure Survival Time	IV								
	IP								
	IM								
	SC		2 [679]						
	PO								

mg/kg		Mouse	Rat	Guinea Pig	Rabbit	Cat	Dog	Monkey	
Decreased Caloric Intake	IV								
	IP								
	IM								
	SC		3 680						
	PO								
Antagonize Reserpine Ptosis	IV								
	IP	12.5 78							
	IM								
	SC								
	PO								
Increased Afferent Vagal Activity	IV					0.05 292	0.05 631		
	IP								
	IM								
	SC								
	PO								
Behavioral	IV								
	IP	50 954							
	IM								
	SC	40 935	5 1050						
	PO								

IN VITRO

mg %	Cardiac	Vascular	Gut	Uterine	Visceral	Skeletal	Trachea	
Rat			0.008 1157	0.012 443				
Guinea Pig			0.02				0.08 1157	
Rabbit	*0.02 67	0.004 1157						
Cat	*0.01 292							

*Total mg

SKF-525-A

(2-Diethylaminoethyl propyldiphenylacetate)

mg/kg		Mouse	Rat	Guinea Pig	Rabbit	Cat	Dog	Monkey	
Lethal Dose $Y-LD_{50}$ $Z-MLD$	IV	Y60 115							
	IP	Y117.5 115	Y163 115						
	IM								
	SC								
	PO	Y538 i15	Y2140 115						
Barbiturate Sleep Potentiation	IV								
	IP	10 681							
	IM								
	SC	50 118							
	PO								
Protects against CCl_4 Toxicity	IV								
	IP		40 1231						
	IM								
	SC								
	PO								
	IV								
	IP								
	IM								
	SC								
	PO								

IN VITRO

mg %	Cardiac	Vascular	Gut	Uterine	Visceral	Skeletal		

SODIUM BROMIDE

(Sedoneural)

mg/kg		Mouse	Rat	Guinea Pig	Rabbit	Cat	Dog	Monkey	
Lethal Dose $Y-LD_{50}$ $Z-MLD$	IV		Z1800 [53]						
	IP								
	IM								
	SC	Y5020 [1063]							
	PO	Y7000 [176]	Y3500 [682]		Z580				
Sedative	IV						350		
	IP								
	IM								
	SC						350		
	PO	3000 [176]			5000	*150 [24]	*1500 [24]		
Anticonvulsant	IV				50				
	IP								
	IM								
	SC	250 [1063]			150				
	PO	2000 [550]							
	IV								
	IP								
	IM								
	SC								
	PO								

*Total dose

IN VITRO

mg %	Cardiac	Vascular	Gut	Uterine	Visceral	Skeletal		

243

SODIUM FLUORIDE

(Florocid, Villiaumite)

mg/kg		Mouse	Rat	Guinea Pig	Rabbit	Cat	Dog	Monkey	
Lethal Dose	IV				87.5 [687]		Z 80 [683]		
Y – LD$_{50}$	IP	125 [109]	Z 31 [683]						
Z – MLD	IM						Z 40 [683]		
	SC	70 [346]	Z 125 [684]	Z 400 [686]		13.7 [109]	155 [109]		
	PO	80 [346]	Y 200 [685]	Z 250 [686]	Z 200 [684]		Z 75 [683]		
	IV								
	IP								
	IM								
	SC								
	PO								
	IV								
	IP								
	IM								
	SC								
	PO								
	IV								
	IP								
	IM								
	SC								
	PO								

IN VITRO

mg %	Cardiac	Vascular	Gut	Uterine	Visceral	Skeletal		

mg/kg		Mouse	Rat	Guinea Pig	Rabbit	Cat	Dog	Monkey	
Lethal Dose $Y-LD_{50}$ $Z-MLD$	IV				Z 85 [689]		Z 15		
	IP								
	IM								
	SC		Z 15 [688]		Z 60 [109]	35 [690]	Z 60 [691]		
	PO						Z 330		
Cardiovascular	IV						10		
	IP		25 [7]						
	IM								
	SC		20 [539]				15		
	PO		40 [7]				*90		
Protect Against Cyanide	IV								
	IP								
	IM		10						
	SC								
	PO								
	IV								
	IP								
	IM								
	SC								
	PO								

*Total dose

IN VITRO

mg %	Cardiac	Vascular	Gut	Uterine	Visceral	Skeletal		
Rabbit		0.01	0.1					

SOTALOL
(MJ-1999)

mg/kg		Mouse	Rat	Guinea Pig	Rabbit	Cat	Dog	Monkey	
Lethal Dose $Y-LD_{50}$ $Z-MLD$	IV								
	IP	Y670 [887]	Y680 [887]				Y330 [887]		
	IM								
	SC								
	PO	Y2600 [887]	Y3450 [887]		Y1000 [887]				
Adrenolytic (α-block)	IV		0.5 [887]						
	IP								
	IM								
	SC		10 [1083]	10 [1081]					
	PO			0.4 [887]			18 [1082]		
Acute Toxicity	IV								
	IP	40 [887]	93 [887]				54 [887]		
	IM								
	SC								
	PO	288 [887]	515 [887]						
	IV								
	IP								
	IM								
	SC								
	PO								

IN VITRO

mg %	Cardiac	Vascular	Gut	Uterine	Visceral	Skeletal		
	10 [1228]							

mg/kg		Mouse	Rat	Guinea Pig	Rabbit	Cat	Dog	Monkey	
Lethal Dose Y—LD$_{50}$ Z—MLD	IV				Z 30 [109]				
	IP								
	IM								
	SC	Z 120 [692]			Z 100 [109]				
	PO								
Cardiovascular	IV				5 [693]	5 [694]	5 [694]		
	IP								
	IM						10 [693]		
	SC						20 [693]		
	PO						60 [693]		
Ganglionic Block	IV					1 [694]			
	IP								
	IM								
	SC								
	PO								
	IV								
	IP								
	IM								
	SC								
	PO								

IN VITRO

mg %	Cardiac	Vascular	Gut	Uterine	Visceral	Skeletal		

STRYCHNINE

mg/kg		Mouse	Rat	Guinea Pig	Rabbit	Cat	Dog	Monkey	
Lethal Dose $Y-LD_{50}$ $Z-MLD$	IV	0.8 [176]	Z1.1 [695]		0.35 [109]	0.33 [109]	0.25 [109]		
	IP	Y0.98 [284]	Y2.1 [696]						
	IM		Z4 [697]						
	SC	Y0.85 [284]	Y1.2 [697]	3.2 [109]	0.7 [109]	0.75 [109]	0.35 [109]		
	PO		Y16.2 [685]		15 [109]	0.75 [109]	1.1 [109]		
Convulsant	IV					0.5 [870]			
	IP	2.5 [924]	1.6 [1220]						
	IM		4						
	SC	1.33	8 [88]		0.4 [611]		0.07		
	PO	2 [935]							
Analeptic	IV				0.6				
	IP								
	IM								
	SC						*0.95 [97]		
	PO					*0.3 [97]	*0.95 [97]		
CNS	IV					0.1 [947]			
	IP					0.1 [1068]			
	IM								
	SC								
	PO								

*Total dose

IN VITRO

mg %	Cardiac	Vascular	Gut	Uterine	Visceral	Skeletal		
Rabbit		1.0	1.0					

SUCCINYLCHOLINE

(Anectine, Quelicin, Suxamethonium)

mg/kg		Mouse	Rat	Guinea Pig	Rabbit	Cat	Dog	Monkey	
Lethal Dose Y−LD50 Z−MLD	IV	Y0.75 111			Y1 281		0.3 281		
	IP	Y4 111							
	IM								
	SC								
	PO	Y125 111							
Neuromuscular Block	IV	0.45 557	0.45 557		0.25 557	0.08 557	0.1		
	IP					1			
	IM								
	SC								
	PO				0.1				
Ataxic and Respiratory (Depression)	IV				0.075				
	IP								
	IM								
	SC						0.05		
	PO								
EEG	IV					0.1 1175			
	IP								
	IM								
	SC								
	PO								

IN VITRO

mg %	Cardiac	Vascular	Gut	Uterine	Visceral	Skeletal		
Rat						0.5 1157		

249

SYROSINGOPINE

(Singoserp, SU-3118)

mg/kg		Mouse	Rat	Guinea Pig	Rabbit	Cat	Dog	Monkey	
Lethal Dose Y–LD$_{50}$ Z–MLD	IV		Y50 640				>3 640	>2 640	
	IP								
	IM								
	SC								
	PO								
Catechol Amine Depletion	IV				1 700	10 836	0.5 700		
	IP	5 698	40 699						
	IM								
	SC								
	PO								
Sedative	IV				4.5 700		5 640	2 640	
	IP		50 699						
	IM								
	SC	25 640							
	PO						> 30 640		
Cardiovascular	IV						1 640		
	IP		0.95 699						
	IM								
	SC								
	PO						3 640		
	IV								
	IP								
	IM								
	SC								
	PO								
	IV								
	IP								
	IM								
	SC								
	PO								

TETRABENAZINE

(Nitoman, RO-1-9569)

mg/kg		Mouse	Rat	Guinea Pig	Rabbit	Cat	Dog	Monkey	
Lethal Dose Y−LD$_{50}$ Z−MLD	IV	Y150 [115]							
	IP								
	IM								
	SC	Y400 [115]							
	PO								
Amine-Depletion	IV				50 [601]	80 [1202]			
	IP	10 [861]	2 [880]						
	IM								
	SC								
	PO								
Barbiturate Sleep Potentiation	IV				50 [601]				
	IP	40 [28]							
	IM								
	SC								
	PO								
Behavioral	IV				40 [703]				
	IP		0.5 [370]						
	IM								
	SC		8 [702]						
	PO								
Sedative	IV								
	IP		20 [899]						
	IM								
	SC							2 [702]	
	PO								
	IV								
	IP								
	IM								
	SC								
	PO								

TETRACAINE

(Amethocaine, Curtacain, Pantocaine)

mg/kg		Mouse	Rat	Guinea Pig	Rabbit	Cat	Dog	Monkey	
Lethal Dose $Y-LD_{50}$ $Z-MLD$	IV	Y70 [7]		Y15.6 [629]	8		Y4.3 [704]		
	IP								
	IM			30 [7]					
	SC								
	PO								
Convulsant	IV		1.5 [705]						
	IP								
	IM								
	SC								
	PO								
Anticonvulsant	IV					0.8			
	IP								
	IM								
	SC	4.4 [441]							
	PO								
	IV								
	IP								
	IM								
	SC								
	PO								

IN VITRO

mg %	Cardiac	Vascular	Gut	Uterine	Visceral	Skeletal		

TETRAETHYLAMMONIUM

(Etamon, TEA)

mg/kg		Mouse	Rat	Guinea Pig	Rabbit	Cat	Dog	Monkey	
Lethal Dose $Y-LD_{50}$ $Z-MLD$	IV	Y29 [214]	Y63 [706]		Y72 [706]		Y55 [706]		
	IP	Y56 [214]	Y115 [706]						
	IM								
	SC	102 [707]							
	PO	Y655 [214]							
Ganglionic Block	IV					10	10		
	IP								
	IM								
	SC								
	PO								
Cardiovascular	IV					3 [708]	5 [708]		
	IP								
	IM								
	SC								
	PO								
EKG	IV					25 [709]	25 [709]		
	IP								
	IM								
	SC								
	PO								
Catechol Amine Sensitization	IV				2.5 [395]	2.5 [395]			
	IP								
	IM								
	SC								
	PO								
Nictitating Membrane Potentiation	IV					2 [395]			
	IP								
	IM								
	SC								
	PO								

TETRAETHYLAMMONIUM (continued)

mg/kg		Mouse	Rat	Guinea Pig	Rabbit	Cat	Dog	Monkey	
Behavioral	IV								
	IP								
	IM								
	SC	80 935							
	PO								
Anticonvulsant	IV								
	IP								
	IM								
	SC	30 957							
	PO								
Decrease Amphetamine Hyperthermia	IV				15 1182				
	IP								
	IM								
	SC								
	PO								
	IV								
	IP								
	IM								
	SC								
	PO								

IN VITRO

mg %	Cardiac	Vascular	Gut	Uterine	Visceral	Skeletal		
Contractile			0.75 388					
Adrenolytic			0.001 395					

mg/kg		Mouse	Rat	Guinea Pig	Rabbit	Cat	Dog	Monkey	
Lethal Dose Y—LD_{50} Z—MLD	IV								
	IP	200 1193							
	IM								
	SC								
	PO								
Cardiovascular	IV					1 1185	6 1189		
	IP								
	IM								
	SC								
	PO								
Behavioral	IV		1 1187						
	IP	25 1198	5 1187						
	IM								
	SC								
	PO		*50 1191					*50 1191	
Hypothermic	IV								
	IP	10 1189							
	IM								
	SC		20 1227						
	PO								
Gastrointestinal	IV								
	IP								
	IM								
	SC	30 1238							
	PO								
	IV								
	IP								
	IM								
	SC								
	PO								

*daily

255

TETRAMETHYLAMMONIUM

(TMA)

mg/kg		Mouse	Rat	Guinea Pig	Rabbit	Cat	Dog	Monkey	
Lethal Dose Y—LD$_{50}$ Z—MLD	IV				1.5 [341]				
	IP								
	IM								
	SC	20 [710]			7 [710]				
	PO								
Ganglionic Stimulant	IV					1	0.25		
	IP								
	IM								
	SC								
	PO								
Decrease Blood Pressure in Experimental Hypertension	IV								
	IP								
	IM								
	SC								
	PO		3 [387]						
	IV								
	IP								
	IM								
	SC								
	PO								

IN VITRO

mg %	Cardiac	Vascular	Gut	Uterine	Visceral	Skeletal		
Guinea Pig	8 [1157]		2 [1157]					

mg/kg		Mouse	Rat	Guinea Pig	Rabbit	Cat	Dog	Monkey	
Lethal Dose Y–LD$_{50}$ Z–MLD	IV								
	IP	>4000 [484]							
	IM								
	SC								
	PO	>5000 [484]							
CNS (Depression)	IV								
	IP	500 [124]	550 [124]				65 [124]		
	IM					100 [557]	300 [557]		
	SC								
	PO	100 [484]		650 [484]					
Anticonvulsant	IV								
	IP	525 [124]							
	IM								
	SC								
	PO								
Decreased Motor Activity	IV								
	IP	1000 [711]							
	IM								
	SC								
	PO	400 [484]		650 [484]					
Barbiturate Sleep Potentiation	IV								
	IP	1000 [711]							
	IM								
	SC								
	PO	1600 [484]							
Block Stress-Induced Ulcer	IV								
	IP								
	IM								
	SC								
	PO	100 [712]							

THALIDOMIDE (continued)

mg/kg		Mouse	Rat	Guinea Pig	Rabbit	Cat	Dog	Monkey	
Potentiate Chlorpromazine and Reserpine Catatonia	IV								
	IP								
	IM								
	SC								
	PO	200 484							
Litter Malformation or Resorption (Fetal Damage)	IV								
	IP								
	IM								
	SC								
	PO		150 859		100 859				
	IV								
	IP								
	IM								
	SC								
	PO								
	IV								
	IP								
	IM								
	SC								
	PO								

IN VITRO

mg %	Cardiac	Vascular	Gut	Uterine	Visceral	Skeletal		
Anticholinergic			3 484					
Antihistiminic			3 484					

258

THEOPHYLLINE

(Acet-Theocin)

mg/kg		Mouse	Rat	Guinea Pig	Rabbit	Cat	Dog	Monkey	
Lethal Dose $Y-LD_{50}$ $Z-MLD$	IV		Z 240		115 [109]				
	IP								
	IM								
	SC	Z 200 [7]	Z 325	185 [109]					
	PO				350 [109]	100 [109]			
Cardiovascular and Diuretic	IV				15	10	20 [898]		
	IP								
	IM								
	SC								
	PO		30						
Increased Motor Activity	IV								
	IP								
	IM								
	SC		20 [180]						
	PO					50 [1007]			
	IV								
	IP								
	IM								
	SC								
	PO								

IN VITRO

mg %	Cardiac	Vascular	Gut	Uterine	Visceral	Skeletal	Trachea	
Antiserotonergic			8.0 [92]					
Guinea Pig							2 [1157]	

THIOPENTAL

(Intraval, Nesdonal, Pentothal)

mg/kg		Mouse	Rat	Guinea Pig	Rabbit	Cat	Dog	Monkey	
Lethal Dose Y−LD$_{50}$ Z−MLD	IV	Y112 713	Y67.5 111	Y55 7	Y40 111		Y55 111		
	IP	Y200 111	Y120 111	Y57.5 714					
	IM								
	SC								
	PO	Y350 111			Y600 111		Y150 111		
Anesthesic	IV	25 111	20 111	20 111	20 111	28 24	25 716		
	IP		40 674	55 111		60 557			
	IM								
	SC								
	PO		70 715				100 111		
Behavioral	IV	17 933			5 562	5 889		0.5−4 1179	
	IP	15 1131							
	IM								
	SC				20 562				
	PO					50 953			
Depressed Spinal Neuron EPSP	IV					40 717			
	IP								
	IM								
	SC								
	PO								
EEG	IV				15 965	20 112	20 966	5 945	
	IP								
	IM								
	SC								
	PO								
Anticonvulsant	IV								
	IP								
	IM								
	SC	30 957							
	PO								

mg/kg		Mouse	Rat	Guinea Pig	Rabbit	Cat	Dog	Monkey	
Lethal Dose $Y-LD_{50}$ $Z-MLD$	IV								
	IP								
	IM								
	SC								
	PO	Y95 [718]							
Sympatholytic	IV					10 [719]			
	IP								
	IM								
	SC								
	PO					17.5 [720]			
Tyramine Potentiation (B.P.)	IV					5			
	IP								
	IM								
	SC								
	PO								
Adrenal Medulla Catechol Amine Depletion	IV								
	IP								
	IM								
	SC		10 [721]						
	PO								

IN VITRO

mg %	Cardiac	Vascular	Gut	Uterine	Visceral	Skeletal		
Adrenolytic [812]			0.5					
Guinea Pig			5 [148]					

β-TM-10

mg/kg		Mouse	Rat	Guinea Pig	Rabbit	Cat	Dog	Monkey	
Lethal Dose Y−LD$_{50}$ Z−MLD	IV	Y6.62 [722]							
	IP								
	IM								
	SC								
	PO	1400 [722]							
Autonomic	IV	4.7 [722]				5 [722]	5 [722]		
	IP								
	IM								
	SC					3 [722]			
	PO					11.3 [720]			
Behavioral	IV								
	IP		30 [722]						
	IM								
	SC								
	PO								
	IV								
	IP								
	IM								
	SC								
	PO								

IN VITRO

mg %	Cardiac	Vascular	Gut	Uterine	Visceral	Skeletal		
Inhibition [812]			10 [722]					

TOLAZOLINE

(Artonil, Priscoline, Vasodil)

mg/kg		Mouse	Rat	Guinea Pig	Rabbit	Cat	Dog	Monkey	
Lethal Dose Y−LD$_{50}$ Z−MLD	IV		67 640						
	IP	Y500							
	IM								
	SC								
	PO								
Adrenolytic	IV	5 1197		1		1	2.5		
	IP	20 1118	10 219	25 1219					
	IM								
	SC								
	PO								
Cardiovascular (Reserpinized)	IV				2 383	1 640	1 640		
	IP								
	IM								
	SC								
	PO								
CNS	IV		15 350						
	IP								
	IM								
	SC								
	PO								

IN VITRO

mg %	Cardiac	Vascular	Gut	Uterine	Visceral	Skeletal		
Rabbit	0.5		1.0					
Rabbit Ear		2 339						
Guinea Pig			0.1 1233					

TRANYLCYPROMINE

(Parnate, SKF-385)

mg/kg		Mouse	Rat	Guinea Pig	Rabbit	Cat	Dog	Monkey	
Lethal Dose Y−LD$_{50}$ Z−MLD	IV	Y37 $_{115}$							
	IP								
	IM								
	SC								
	PO	Y38 $_{115}$							
Increased Catechol Amines (Brain)	IV				5 $_{371}$				
	IP	10 $_{433}$	2 $_{1064}$						
	IM		4 $_{1064}$						
	SC		3 $_{868}$						
	PO		5 $_{433}$						
Reverse Reserpine Depression	IV								
	IP	2.5 $_{455}$							
	IM								
	SC								
	PO	2.5 $_{455}$							
EEG	IV				2 $_{331}$		2 $_{1006}$		
	IP								
	IM								
	SC								
	PO								
Cardiovascular	IV		5 $_{218}$						
	IP								
	IM								
	SC								
	PO								
CNS Stimulation and Behavioral	IV					15 $_{861}$	4 $_{160}$		
	IP	5 $_{1064}$							
	IM								
	SC								
	PO								

mg/kg		Mouse	Rat	Guinea Pig	Rabbit	Cat	Dog	Monkey	
Lethal Dose Y—LD$_{50}$ Z—MLD	IV								
	IP								
	IM								
	SC								
	PO								
Tremor and Decreased Brain Amines	IV	20 [723]	5-20 [724]	5-20 [724]		5-20 [724]	5-20 [724]	5-20 [724]	
	IP	5-20 [724]	5-20 [724]	20 [724]		5-20 [724]	5 [723]	5-20 [724]	
	IM	5-20 [724]	5-20 [724]	5-20 [724]		5-20 [724]	5-20 [724]	5-20 [724]	
	SC	20 [76]	5-20 [724]	5-20 [724]		5-20 [724]	5-20 [724]	5-20 [724]	
	PO	20 [723]	5-20 [724]	5-20 [724]		5-20 [724]	5-20 [724]	5-20 [724]	
Increased Brain Histamine	IV								
	IP								
	IM								
	SC		100						
	PO								
Convulsant	IV								
	IP	5.8 [139]							
	IM								
	SC								
	PO								
Analgetic	IV								
	IP								
	IM	5							
	SC	6 [1066]							
	PO								
EEG	IV								
	IP					3 [725]			
	IM								
	SC								
	PO								

TRIBROMOETHANOL

(Avertin, Bromethol, Narcolan)

mg/kg		Mouse	Rat	Guinea Pig	Rabbit	Cat	Dog	Monkey	
Lethal Dose Y−LD$_{50}$ Z−MLD	IV				135 [66]	300 [557]	300 [557]		
	IP	600 [66]	550 [726]		400 [66]				
	IM								
	SC	500 [66]	730 [727]						
	PO		1000 [728]		2000 [109]	150 [66]			
Anesthetic	IV	120 [66]		100 [66]	80 [66]	100 [557]	125 [557]		
	IP	250 [200]	550 [547]		225 [66]				
	IM		400 [547]						
	SC				500 [66]				
	PO				600 [66]	100 [66]			
	IV								
	IP								
	IM								
	SC								
	PO								
	IV								
	IP								
	IM								
	SC								
	PO								

IN VITRO

mg %	Cardiac	Vascular	Gut	Uterine	Visceral	Skeletal		

TRIFLUOPERAZINE

(Eskazine, Stelazine, Terfluzine)

mg/kg		Mouse	Rat	Guinea Pig	Rabbit	Cat	Dog	Monkey	
Lethal Dose $Y-LD_{50}$ $Z-MLD$	IV	Y36 [82]					Y60 [82]		
	IP								
	IM								
	SC								
	PO	Y442 [82]	Y740 [82]						
Behavior	IV								
	IP		1 [577]						
	IM			0.3 [1053]				0.25 [1053]	
	SC		0.43 [95]						
	PO	1 [729]	12.8 [1056]						
Catatonic	IV								
	IP		165 [227]						
	IM								
	SC								
	PO	25 [730]	2.6 [730]				10 [1041]	20 [730]	
Decreased Spontaneous Motor Activity	IV								
	IP								
	IM								
	SC								
	PO	10 [730]	2.5 [730]					10 [730]	
Barbiturate Sleep Potentiation	IV								
	IP	1 [227]							
	IM								
	SC								
	PO								
EEG	IV				2 [824]				
	IP								
	IM								
	SC								
	PO								

TRIMETHADIONE

(Tridione, Trimedone, Trimetin)

mg/kg		Mouse	Rat	Guinea Pig	Rabbit	Cat	Dog	Monkey	
Lethal Dose Y—LD$_{50}$ Z—MLD	IV	Y2000 [731]			Y1500 [731]				
	IP	Y1800 [111]			Y1500 [731]				
	IM								
	SC		Y2200 [111]						
	PO	Y2200 [111]							
Anticonvulsant	IV	275 [881]	200 [111]						
	IP	150 [592]	300 [111]		500				
	IM							50 [1096]	
	SC	225			500				
	PO	400	70 [1038]		942 [1012]	30 [97]	30 [97]		
Hypnotic	IV	1500			750 [111]				
	IP	1500							
	IM								
	SC		1500 [63]						
	PO	1500							
Behavioral	IV								
	IP								
	IM								
	SC								
	PO	800 [935]							
EEG	IV				200 [1223]	500 [1222]			
	IP								
	IM								
	SC								
	PO								
	IV								
	IP								
	IM								
	SC								
	PO								

TRIPELENNAMINE

(Dehistin, Pyribenzamine, Tonaril)

mg/kg		Mouse	Rat	Guinea Pig	Rabbit	Cat	Dog	Monkey	
Lethal Dose Y—LD$_{50}$ Z—MLD	IV	Y17 [732]	Y13 [732]		9		42.7		
	IP	Y70 [732]							
	IM								
	SC	Y75 [324]	Y225 [324]	Y30.2 [221]	33 [324]				
	PO	Y210 [324]	Y570 [324]	Y155 [221]					
Antihistaminic	IV			19 [221]		5.5 [97]	5.5 [97]		
	IP			10					
	IM			5					
	SC			5					
	PO			5.3 [648]		5.5 [97]	5.5 [97]		
Cardiovascular Potentiation of Aldehydes and Norepinephrine	IV		*2.5 [1074]			2 [496]	4 [263]		
	IP								
	IM								
	SC								
	PO								
Behavioral	IV								
	IP		5.2 [848]						
	IM								
	SC								
	PO								

*Total dose

IN VITRO

mg %	Cardiac	Vascular	Gut	Uterine	Visceral	Skeletal		
Antiserotonergic			0.1 [92]					
Antihistaminic			0.005 [93]					
Anticholinergic			6 [93]					

TUBOCURARINE

(Delacurarin, Tubadil, Tubarine)

mg/kg		Mouse	Rat	Guinea Pig	Rabbit	Cat	Dog	Monkey	
Lethal Dose Y−LD$_{50}$ Z−MLD	IV	0.14 733		0.1 736	Y0.35 735		3		
	IP	Y0.14 734	Y0.25 735						
	IM						10 111		
	SC	0.53 733	0.3	0.1 109	0.34 109	0.34 109	0.34 109		
	PO								
Neuromuscular Block	IV	0.075 736	0.075 736	0.035 736	0.12 735	0.15	0.1	0.75 442	
	IP								
	IM				0.4 736	0.7 557	0.15		
	SC				0.5 361		0.15		
	PO								
Cardiovascular	IV					0.1 736	0.1 736		
	IP								
	IM								
	SC								
	PO								
CNS	IV		0.05 1000			0.05 1000			
	IP								
	IM								
	SC								
	PO								

IN VITRO

mg %	Cardiac	Vascular	Gut	Uterine	Visceral	Skeletal		
Rat						0.05 1157		
Rabbit	0.1		0.1					

mg/kg		Mouse	Rat	Guinea Pig	Rabbit	Cat	Dog	Monkey	
Lethal Dose	IV				300 [109]				
$Y-LD_{50}$	IP								
$Z-MLD$	IM								
	SC	225 [109]				30 [109]			
	PO								
Cardiovascular	IV		0.1		0.1	0.5	0.25 [408]		
	IP								
	IM								
	SC	30 [737]							
	PO								
Decreased Tissue Uptake of Norepinephrine	IV					10 [91]			
	IP	80 [338]							
	IM		20 [738]						
	SC								
	PO								
Amine-Depletion	IV	5 [861]							
	IP		20 [879]						
	IM								
	SC								
	PO								

IN VITRO

mg %	Cardiac	Vascular	Gut	Uterine	Visceral	Skeletal		
Rat	0.002 [301]			0.17 [1157]				
Ear—Rabbit		*0.016 [339]						
Langendorff	*0.01 [739]							

*Total mg

URETHAN(E)

(Ethyl Carbamate)

mg/kg		Mouse	Rat	Guinea Pig	Rabbit	Cat	Dog	Monkey	
Lethal Dose Y−LD_{50} Z−MLD	IV				2000				
	IP	Z 2150 194							
	IM								
	SC		1800						
	PO						2500		
Anesthetic	IV				1000	1250	1000 413		
	IP		780 127	1500	1000	1500			
	IM		950 166			1800	1000		
	SC		950 166		1500	1000 740			
	PO					750	1500 550		
Sedative	IV								
	IP								
	IM								
	SC								
	PO	400 935				*1250 97	*1250 97		
Increase Acetylcholine (Brain)	IV								
	IP		1000 1209						
	IM								
	SC								
	PO								

*Total dose

IN VITRO

mg %	Cardiac	Vascular	Gut	Uterine	Visceral	Skeletal		

mg/kg		Mouse	Rat	Guinea Pig	Rabbit	Cat	Dog	Monkey	
Lethal Dose Y−LD$_{50}$ Z−MLD	IV	Y0.42 [639]							
	IP	Y1.35 [640]	Y3.5 [639]						
	IM								
	SC								
	PO								
Cardiovascular	IV					*0.07 [741]	0.005 [742]		
	IP								
	IM								
	SC								
	PO								
Respiratory (Depression)	IV								
	IP						0.6 [643]		
	IM								
	SC								
	PO								
	IV								
	IP								
	IM								
	SC								
	PO								

*Total dose

IN VITRO

mg %	Cardiac	Vascular	Gut	Uterine	Visceral	Skeletal		

WARFARIN

(Coumadin, Maveran, Prothromadin)

mg/kg		Mouse	Rat	Guinea Pig	Rabbit	Cat	Dog	Monkey	
Lethal Dose Y−LD$_{50}$ Z−MLD	IV	Y165 [111]	Y186 [743]		Y150 [743]		Y250 [743]		
	IP								
	IM								
	SC								
	PO	Y374 [743]	Y323 [743]	Y182 [743]	Y800 [743]		Y250 [743]		
	IV								
	IP								
	IM								
	SC								
	PO								
	IV								
	IP								
	IM								
	SC								
	PO								
	IV								
	IP								
	IM								
	SC								
	PO								

IN VITRO

mg %	Cardiac	Vascular	Gut	Uterine	Visceral	Skeletal		
Ionotropic (Negative)	25 [744]							

YOHIMBINE

(Aphrodine, Corynine, Quebrachine)

mg/kg		Mouse	Rat	Guinea Pig	Rabbit	Cat	Dog	Monkey	
Lethal Dose Y—LD$_{50}$ Z—MLD	IV	16 [745]			11 [109]				
	IP								
	IM								
	SC				50 [109]		20 [346]		
	PO	40 [346]							
Adrenolytic	IV		5		2		0.2 [746]		
	IP								
	IM								
	SC								
	PO								
CNS	IV				8 [1067]				
	IP	5 [350]							
	IM								
	SC		5 [350]						
	PO								
	IV								
	IP								
	IM								
	SC								
	PO								

IN VITRO

mg %	Cardiac	Vascular	Gut	Uterine	Visceral	Skeletal		
Antiserotonergic			0.5 [92]					

ZOXAZOLAMINE

(Flexin, McN-485, Contrazole)

mg/kg		Mouse	Rat	Guinea Pig	Rabbit	Cat	Dog	Monkey	
Lethal Dose	IV						Y117 [1176]		
Y−LD$_{50}$	IP	Y376 [461]	Y102 [461]						
Z−MLD	IM								
	SC								
	PO	Y825 [461]	Y376 [461]						
Loss of Righting Reflex	IV						37 [1176]		
	IP	81 [461]	43 [461]						
	IM								
	SC								
	PO	415 [461]	137 [461]						
Decrease Decerebrate Rigidity	IV					30 [191]			
	IP								
	IM								
	SC								
	PO	120 [191]							
Crossed- Extensor Reflex Depressant	IV					60			
	IP								
	IM								
	SC								
	PO								
Antistrychnine	IV								
	IP	227 [461]							
	IM								
	SC								
	PO	120 [1016]							
Behavioral and EEG	IV					60 [1016]			
	IP								
	IM								
	SC								
	PO	200 [935]							

APPENDIX A

HORMONE MAINTENANCE AND REPLACEMENT DOSAGE

Species	Effect of Hormone	Dose	Route	Reference
	Hypophysectomized			
Mouse	Double Uterine Weight			
	Pregnant mare's serum gonadotrophin	1.8 IU	SC	754
Rat	Restore spermatogenesis			
	Testosterone propionate	3 mg/day/35 days	IP	755
	Stimulate ovarian growth			
	Diethylstilbestrol	1 mg/day/8 days	SC	756
	Estradiol	1 mg/day/8 days	SC	756
	Restore fatty acid synthesis			
	Thyroxine	0.1 mg/kg/day	IP	757
	ACTH	0.05 mg/day/14 days	IP	758
	Return O_2 consumption to normal			
	Thyroxine	0.01 mg/day	SC	759
	Corticosterone	1 mg/day/14 days	SC	760
	Cortisone Acetate	1 mg/day/14 days	SC	760
	Hydrocortisone Acetate	1 mg/day/14 days	SC	760
	Increase body weight to normal			
	Somatotropin	0.125 ⎫	SC	761
	(plus) Corticosterone	0.015 ⎬ mg/halfday		
	(and) Thyroxine	0.003 ⎭		
Dog	Restore normal carbohydrate metabolism			
	Cortisone	1 mg/kg/day	IM	762
	Hydrocortisone	1 mg/kg/day	IM	762
	Produce hyperthyroid state			
	Thyroxin	0.4 mg/kg/day	IM	762
	Pancreatectomized			
Rat	Maintain weight			
	Insulin	1 unit/halfday	SC	763
	Maintain glucosurea			
	Insulin	18 units/day	SC	764
	Maintain serum gamma globulin during stress			
	Insulin	0.033 unit/halfday	SC	765
	Exacerbation of urinary glucose			
	Progesterone	50 mg/day	SC	766
	11-Desoxycorticosterone acetate	10 mg/day	SC	767

HORMONE MAINTENANCE AND REPLACEMENT DOSAGE

Species	Effect of Hormone	Dose	Route	Reference
	Pancreatectomized (continued)			
Rabbit	Maintain weight on carbohydrate diet			
	Insulin	12 units/day	SC	768
Dog	Decrease glucose content of blood			
	Testosterone propionate	40 mg	IM	769
Baboon	Control diabetes			
	Insulin	2.5 units/kg/day	IV	770
	Adrenalectomized			
Rat	Maintenance dose			
	Hydrocortisone	0.1 mg/halfday	SC	771
	Cortexone acetate	0.1 mg/day	SC	772
	Diethylstilbestrol	0.1 mg/day	SC	773
	Return blood sugar to normal			
	Aldosterone	0.1 mg/day/9 days	SC	774
	Hydrocortisone acetate	15 mg/day/3 days	SC	775
	Return spontaneous activity to normal			
	Cortisone	5 mg/day/10 days	SC, PO	776
	Hydrocortisone	5 mg/day/10 days	SC	777
	Restore normal metabolism in adipose tissue			
	Dexamethasone	10 µg	IP	778
	Increase blood protein			
	Aldosterone	0.1 mg/day/12 days	SC	779
	Return plasma Na to normal			
	Aldosterone acetate	0.5 mg/kg	SC	780
	Block increase in antibody formation			
	Cortisone	80 mg/kg	SC	781
	Decrease heat loss on exposure to cold			
	Cortisone	1 mg/day	SC	782
	Adrenal cortical extract	0.25 mg/day	SC	782
	Prevent involution of pancreas acinar cells			
	Cortisone	0.5 mg/halfday	SC	783
Guinea Pig	Maintenance dose			
	Deoxycorticosterone	1 mg/day	SC	784
	Anesthetic dose			
	Deoxycortisone glucoside	100 mg	SC	784
Cat	Retard salivary gland atrophy			
	Deoxycorticosterone	5.0 mg/kg/day	SC	782
Dog	Maintenance dose			
	Cortisone acetate	25 mg/day	PO }	785
	(plus) Desoxycosticosterone acetate-1	2 mg/day	IM }	
	Desoxycorticosterone acetate	2.5 mg/day	IM	762
Monkey		Maintenance dose	50 mg/day x 1	IM	
	Hydrocortisone sodium succinate	20 mg/day x 3	IM	
		10 mg/day (cont'd)	IM	1079

HORMONE MAINTENANCE AND REPLACEMENT DOSAGE

Species	Effect of Hormone	Dose	Route	Reference
	Castrated			
Mouse	Maintenance dose			
	Testosterone phenylacetate	1.0 mg/10 days	SC	249
	Produce female-like mammary develop-ment			
	Estrone	92.5 µg	SC	786
Rat	Maintenance dose			
	Testosterone phenylacetate	50 mg/kg	SC	787
	Increase weight of seminal vesicles			
	Testosterone	0.4 mg/day/7 days	SC	788
	Testosterone	1.0 mg/day/7 days	IP, PO	788
	Testosterone propionate	0.5 mg/day/20 days	SC	789
	Testosterone propionate	0.4 mg/day/7 days	IP	788
	Testosterone propionate	1.0 mg/day/7 days	PO	788
	Methyltestosterone	0.4 mg/day/7 days	SC, IP, PO	788
	Inhibit calcium loss			
	Testosterone	2 mg/day	SC	790
	Return of spontaneous activity to normal			
	Testosterone propionate	20 mg/day/10 days	SC	776
	Prevent prostatic epithelial cell atrophy			
	Testosterone	100 µg/kg/day	SC	791
Guinea Pig	Return seminal vesicle weight and metabolism to normal			
	Testosterone propionate	2 mg/day	SC	792
	Diminish the fall in hepatic glycogen			
	Testosterone	15 mg/2 days/30 days	SC	793
	Decrease nondirected hyperexcitability			
	Testosterone	250 µg/kg/day	SC	794
	Ovariectomized			
Mice	Induce mammary growth in immature			
	Estrone	0.006 µg/day/21 days	SC	795
Rat	Hormone replacement			
	Estradiol benzoate	0.015 mg/kg/day	SC	796
	Polyestradiol phosphate	20 mg/kg/day	SC	787
	Increase vaginal cornification and activity			
	Dienestral	1 ⎫	PO, SC	776
	Hexestral	1 ⎪	SC	776
	Hexestral	40 ⎬ µg/day/10 days	PO	776
	Stilbestrol	1 ⎪	SC	776
	Stilbestrol	4 ⎭	PO	776
	Pregnancy maintenance			
	Acetonide	10 mg/day	SC, PO	797
	Acetophenone	20 mg/day	SC, PO	797
	Progesterone	20 mg/day	SC, PO	797
	Return spontaneous activity to normal			
	Estrone benzoate	1 mg/day/10 days	SC	776
	Lower ECS threshold			
	Estradiol	5 mg/kg/day/7 days	SC	798

HORMONE MAINTENANCE AND REPLACEMENT DOSAGE

Species	Effect of Hormone	Dose	Route	Reference
	Thyroidectomized			
Rat	Maintenance dose			
	Thyroxine	0.005 mg/day	IP	799
	Return metabolic rate to normal			
	Thyroxine	0.015 mg/kg/day	IP	800
	Improve or normalize glucose tolerance			
	Triiodothyroxine	0.02 mg/day/4 days	SC	801
Guinea Pig	Increase metabolism			
	Thyrotropic hormone	25 units/day/12 days	IM	802
	Thyroparathyroidectomized			
Rat	Replacement therapy in lactating female			
	Thyroxin	30 μg/kg/day	SC	
	(plus) Parathyroid hormone	300 USPU/kg/day	SC	803
	Produce arthritis			
	Deoxycorticosterone acetate	2 mg/day	SC	804
Dog	Return intestinal Ca absorption to normal			
	Parathyroid extract	500 IU	IV	805
	Parathyroidectomized			
Rat	Increase excretion of urinary phosphate			
	Parathyroid hormone	20 USPU	SC	806
	Parathyroid hormone	1.0 IU/hour	SC	807
	Cortisone	10 mg/day	IP	808

APPENDIX B

PHYSIOLOGICAL SOLUTIONS
(Gm/liter)

	NaCl	KCl	$CaCl_2$	$MgCl_2$	$NaHCO_3$	NaH_2PO_4	KH_2PO_4	$MgSO_4$	Glucose
Saline (Mammal)	9.00	--	--	--	--	--	--	--	--
Ringer (Mammal)	9.00	0.42	0.24	--	0.50	--	--	--	1.00
Ringer (by Cattell)	9.00	0.42	0.12	--	--	--	0.100	--	1.00
Ringer (by Dresel)	6.00	0.531	0.35	--	2.10	--	0.081	0.147	0.90
Ringer (by Evans)	--	0.42	0.12	0.200	--	--	--	--	1.00[a, b]
Ringer (by Genell)	8.00	0.42	0.24	0.005	1.00	--	--	--	0.50
Ringer (by Moran)	7.00	0.42	0.24	0.200	2.10	--	--	--	1.80
Ringer-Dale (by Stewart)	9.00	0.42	2.015	0.003	0.50	--	--	--	0.50
Ringer-Locke (same as Locke's)	9.00	0.42	0.24	--	0.15	--	--	--	1.75
Ringer-Locke (by Feldberg)	9.00	0.20	0.20	--	0.30	--	--	--	1.00
Ringer-Locke (by Gaddum)	9.00	0.42	0.06	--	0.50	--	--	--	0.50
Ringer-Locke (by Hukovic)	9.00	0.42	0.24	--	0.50	--	--	--	2.00
Locke's (by Burn)	9.00	0.42	0.24	0.005	0.50	--	--	--	0.50
Krebs-Henseleit	6.87	0.40	0.28	--	2.10	0.140	--	0.140	2.00
Krebs-Henseleit-Ringer	6.90	0.354	0.280	--	2.10	--	0.162	0.294	--
Krebs-Henseleit (by Furchgott)	6.90	0.354	0.282	--	2.10	--	0.162	0.294	1.80
Krebs (by Hukovic)	6.60	0.350	0.280	--	2.10	--	0.162	0.294	2.08
Beauvilain's	9.00	0.42	0.06	0.005	0.50	--	--	--	0.50
McEwan's	7.60	0.42	0.24	--	2.10	0.143	--	--	2.00[c]
Tyrode (Isolated Gut)	8.00	0.20	0.20	0.100	1.00	0.050	--	--	1.00
Feigen's (Isolated Heart)	9.00	0.42	0.62	--	0.60	--	--	--	1.00

[a] K_2SO_4 = 22.00   [b] $KHCO_3$ = 3.60   [c] Sucrose = 4.50

BIBLIOGRAPHY

1. Skog, E. A Toxicological Investigation of Lower Aliphatic Aldehydes. I. Toxicity of Formaldehyde, Acetaldehyde, Propionaldehyde and Butyraldehyde; as well as of Acrolein and Crotonaldehyde. Acta pharmacol. (Kbh.) 6: 299-318, 1950.

2. Stotz, E., et al. Behavioral and Pharmacological Studies of Thiopropazate, a Potent Tranquilizing Agent. Arch. int. Pharmacodyn. 127:85-103, 1960.

3. Supniewski, J. V. The Toxic Action of Acetaldehyde on the Organs of Vertebrata. J. Pharmacol. exp. Ther. 30:429-437, 1927.

4. Sollmann, T. H. and P. J. Hanzlik. Fundamentals of Experimental Pharmacology. J. W. Stacey, Inc., San Francisco, 1940.

5. Eade, N. R. Mechanism of Sympathomimetic Action of Aldehydes. J. Pharmacol. exp. Ther. 127:29-34, 1959.

6. Kreitmair, D. H. The Pharmacological Action of Ephedrine. Arch. exp. Path. Pharmakol. 120:189-228, 1927.

7. Anderson, H. H., et al. Pharmacology and Experimental Therapeutics. University of California Press, Berkeley and Los Angeles, 1947.

8. Smith, P. K. and W. E. Hambourger. The Ratio of the Toxicity of Acetanilid to its Antipyretic Activity in Rats. J. Pharmacol. exp. Ther. 54:159-160, 1935.

9. Smith, P. K. and W. E. Hambourger. The Ratio of the Toxicity of Acetanilide and its Antipyretic Activity in Rats. J. Pharmacol. exp. Ther. 54:346-351, 1935.

10. Lester, D. Formation of Methemoglobin. J. Pharmacol. exp. Ther. 77:154-159, 1943.

11. Munch, J. C., et al. Acetanilid Studies. I. Acute Toxicity. J. Amer. pharm. Ass. 30:91-98, 1941.

12. Karczmar, A. G. The Effects of Lethal Doses of Acetanilid in the Dog. Fed. Proc. 6:341-343, 1947.

13. Molitor, H. A Comparative Study of the Effects of Five Choline Compounds Used in Therapeutics: Acetylcholine Chloride, Acetyl Beta-Methylcholine Chloride, Carbaminoyl Choline, Ethyl Ether Beta-Methyl-choline Chloride, Carbaminoyl Beta-Methylcholine Chloride. J. Pharmacol. exp. Ther. 58: 337-360, 1936.

14. Monnier, M. Electro-Physiological Actions of Central Nervous System Stimulants. Arch. int. Pharmacodyn. 124:281-301, 1960.

15. Trendelenburg, U. and J. S. Gravenstein. Effect of Reserpine Pretreatment on Stimulation of the Accelerans Nerve of the Dog. Science 128:901-902, 1958.

16. Fraser, P. J. Pharmacologic Actions of Pure Muscarine Chloride. Brit. J. Pharmacol. 12:47-52, 1957.

17. Ben-Bassat, J., et al. Analgesimetry and Ranking of Analgesic Drugs by the Receptacle Method. Arch. int. Pharmacodyn. 122:434-447, 1959.

18. Hart, E. R. The Toxicity and Analgetic Potency of Salicylamide and Certain of its Derivatives as Compared with Established Analgetic-Antipyretic Drugs. J. Pharmacol. exp. Ther. 89:205-209, 1947.

19. Ichniowski, C. T. and W. C. Hueper, Pharmacological and Toxicological Studies on Salicylamide. J. Am. pharm. Ass. 35: 225-230, 1946.

20. Eagle, E. and A. J. Carlson. Toxicity, Antipyretic and Analgesic Studies on 39 Compounds Including Aspirin, Phenacetin and 27 Derivatives of Carbazole and Tetrahydrocarbazole. J. Pharmacol. exp. Ther. 99:450-457, 1950.

21. Smith, C. S., et al. The Analgesic Properties of Certain Drugs and Drug Combinations. J. Pharmacol. exp. Ther. 77:184-193, 1943.

22. Winder, C. V. Quantitative Evaluation of Analgesic Action in Guinea Pigs. Morphine, Ethyl 1-Methyl-4-Phenylpiperidine-4-Carboxylate (Demerol) and Acetylsalicylic Acid. Arch. int. Pharmacodyn. 74:219-226, 1947.

23. Eillinger, A. Aromatic Hydrocarbons, Phenols, Aromatic Acids, Aromatic Alcohols, Aldehydes, Ketones, Quinines and Nitro Compounds. Heffter's Hdb. 1:871-1048, 1923.

24. Jones, L. M. Veterinary Pharmacology and Therapeutics. The Iowa State College Press, Ames, Iowa, 1957.

25. Guerra, F. and G. H. Barbour. The Mechanism of Aspirin Antipyresis in Monkeys. J. Pharmacol. exp. Ther. 79:55-61, 1943.

26. Collier, H. O. J., et al. The Bronchoconstrictor Action of Bradykinin in the Guinea Pig. Brit. J. Pharmacol. 15:290-297, 1960.

27. Launey, L. Determination of Toxicity and Activity of Several Barbiturate Derivatives. Principles of Comparison. J. Physiol. Path. gén. 30:364-378, 1932.

28. Pletscher, A., et al. Bensoquinolizine, a New Compound with an Action on 5-Hydroxytryptamine and Norepinephrine in the Brain. Arch. exp. Path. Pharmakol. 232:499-509, 1958.

29. Barlow, O. W. Studies on the Pharmacology of Ethyl Alcohol. I. A Comparative Study of the Pharmacologic Effects of Grain and Synthetic Ethyl Alcohols. II. A Correlation of the Local Irritant, Anesthetic and Toxic Effects of Three Potable Whiskeys with their Alcoholic Content. J. Pharmacol. exp. Ther. 56:117-146, 1936.

30. Alekseeva, I. A. The Direct and Conditioned Reflex Effects of Inhibitory Substances on the Higher Nervous Activity of Dogs with Organic Lesions of Certain Parts of the Cerebral Cortex. Pavlov J. higher nerv. Activ. 10:737-744, 1960.

31. Bonnycastle, D. D., et al. The Effect of a Number of Central Depressant Drugs upon Brain 5-Hydroxytryptamine Levels in the Rat. J. Pharmacol. exp. Ther. 135:17-20, 1962.

32. Miller, N. E. and H. Barry. Motivational Effects of Drugs: Some General Problems in Psychopharmacology. Psychopharmacologia 1:169-199, 1960.

33. Lehman, A. J. Chemicals in Food: A Report to the Association of Food and Drug Officials on Current Developments. Assoc. Food & Drug Officials U. S. Quart. Bull. 15:122-133, 1951.

34. Witkin, L. B., et al. A Study of Some Central Stimulants in Mice. Arch. int. Pharmacodyn. 124:105-115, 1960.

35. Hanzlik, P. J., et al. Toxicity, Fats and Excretion of Propylene Glycol and Some Other Glycols. J. Pharmacol. exp. Ther. 67:101-126, 1939.

36. Waisbren, B. A. Alloxan Diabetes in Mice. Proc. Soc. exp. Biol. (N.Y.) 67:154-156, 1948.

37. Gabe, M. Histological Changes of the Liver and Heart Following Acute Alloxan Intoxication in the Albino Rat. C. R. Soc. Biol. (Paris) 142:1335-1340, 1948.

38. Lazarow, A. Protective Effect of Glutathione against Alloxan Diabetes in the Rat. Proc. Soc. exp. Biol. (N.Y.) 61:441-447, 1946.

39. Gomeri, G. and M. G. Goldner. Production of Diabetes Mellitus in Rats with Alloxan. Proc. Soc. exp. Biol. (N.Y.) 54:287-290, 1943.

40. Duff, G. L. and H. Starr. Experimental Alloxan Diabetes in Hooded Rats. Proc. Soc. exp. Biol. (N.Y.) 57:280-282, 1944.

41. Goldner, M. G. and G. Gomori. Alloxan Diabetes in the Dog. Endocrinology 33:297-308, 1943.

42. Gruber, C. M., et al. Studies on the Pharmacology and Toxicology of dl-α-1,3-Dimethyl-4-Phenyl-4-Propionoxy Piperidine (Nu-1196). J. Pharmacol. exp. Ther. 99:312-316, 1950.

43. Randall, L. O. and G. Lehman. Pharmacological Properties of Some Neostigmine Analogs. J. Pharmacol. exp. Ther. 99:16-32, 1950.

44. Maney, P. V., et al. Dihydroxypropyltheophylline: Its Preparation and Pharmacological

Clinical Study. J. Amer. pharm. Ass., sci. Ed. 35:266-272, 1946.

45. Thompson, C. R. and M. R. Warren. Acute and Chronic Toxicity Studies on Theophylline Aminoisobutanol and Theophylline Ethylenediamine. J. Lab. clin. Med. 31:1337-1343, 1946.

46. Warecka, K. The Influence of Euphylline, Chlorpromazine and Reserpine on the Pia Mater Blood Vessels of Cats and Rabbits. Acta physiol. pharmacol. neerl. 9:452-460, 1960.

47. Christensen, J. M., et al. Ethylnorephrine: A Unique Bronchodilator. Amer. Practit. 9: 916-921, 1958.

48. Cameron, W. M., et al. Further Evidences on the Nature of the Vasomotor Actions of Ethylnorsuprarenin. J. Pharmacol. exp. Ther. 63:340-351, 1938.

49. Koch, R. On the Toxicity of Pyramidon. Med. Klin. 45:661-665, 1950.

50. Domenjoz, R. The Pharmacology of Phenylbutazone Analogues. Ann. N.Y. Acad. Sci. 86: 263, 1960.

51. Rose, C. L. Detoxification of Amidopyrine by Sodium Amytal. Proc. Soc. exp. Biol. (N.Y.) 32:1242-1243, 1935.

52. Hazelton, L. W., et al. Acute and Chronic Toxicity of Butazolidin. J. Pharmacol. exp. Ther. 109:387-392, 1953.

53. Loeser, D. and A. L. Konwiser. A Study of the Toxicity of Strontium and Comparison with Other Cations Employed in Therapeutics. J. Lab. clin. Med. 15:35-41, 1929.

54. Horwitt, M. K., et al. Heat Regulation and Water Exchange. J. Pharmacol. exp. Ther. 48:217-222, 1933.

55. Winder, C. V., et al. A Study of Pharmacological Influences on Ultraviolet Erythema in Guinea Pigs. Arch. int. Pharmacodyn. 116: 261, 1958.

56. Filehne, W. Pyramidon. Z. klin. Med. 32: 569-577, 1897.

57. Biberfeld, J. Pharmacological Studies on Some Pyrazolon Derivatives. Zschr. exp. Path. 5:28-42, 1908.

58. Merck Institute. Personal Communication

59. Herr, F. et al. Tranquilizers and Antidepressants: A Pharmacological Comparison. Arch. int. Pharmacodyn. 134:328-342, 1961.

60. Steiner, W. G. and H. E. Himwich. Central Cholinolytic Action of Chlorpromazine. Science 136:873-875, 1962.

61. Feldman, S. A. Effect of Decamethonium upon Conditioned Reflexes in Rats. Anaesthesia 15:55-60, 1960.

62. Amberg, S. and H. F. Helmholz. The Fatal Dose of Various Substances on Intravenous Injection in the Guinea Pig. J. Pharmacol. exp. Ther. 6:595, 1915.

63. Swanson, E. E. and W. E. Fry. A Comparative Study of Two Short Acting Barbituric Acid Derivatives. J. Amer. pharm. Ass. 26:1248-1249, 1937.

64. Holck, H. G. and M. A. Kanan. Intravenous Lethal Doses of Amytal in the Dog and Rabbit and a Table of Animal Dosages Compiled from the Literature. J. Lab. clin. Med. 19: 1191-1205, 1934.

65. Butler, T. C. The Delay in Onset of Intravenously Injected Anesthetics. J. Pharmacol. exp. Ther. 74:118-128, 1942.

66. Heubner, W. and J. Schuller. Narcotics of the Aliphatic Series. Heffter's Hdb. E. 2:1-282, 1936.

67. Hirschfelder, A. D. and R. N. Bieter. Local Anesthetics. Physiol. Rev. 12:190-282, 1932.

68. Vogt, M. Comparative Studies in Circulatory Damage and Narcotic Effect of Various Barbituric Acid Derivatives. Arch exp. Path. Pharmakol. 152:341-360, 1930.

69. Swett, L. R., et al. Structure-Activity Relations in the Pargyline Series. Ann. N.Y. Acad. Sci. 107:891-898, 1963.

70. Gruber, C. M., et al. III. The Toxic Actions of Sodium Diphenyl Hydantoinate (Dilantin) when Injected Intraperitoneally and Intravenously in Experimental Animals. J. Pharmacol. exp. Ther. 68:433-436, 1940.

71. Maloney, A. H. Picrotoxin as an Antidote in Acute Poisoning by the Barbiturates. J. Pharmacol. exp. Ther. 42:267-268, 1931.

72. Gruber, C. M. and G. F. Keyser. A Study on the Development of Tolerance and Cross

Tolerance to Barbiturates in Experimental Animals. J. Phramacol. exp. Ther. 86:186-196, 1946.

73. Halpern, B. N. Toxicity and Cardiovascular Action of β-Phenylisopropylamine (Benzedrine). J. Physiol. Path. gén. 37:597-614, 1939.

74. Heubner, W. and M. Stuhlman. A Notice on Benzedrine and Pervitin. Arch. exp. Path. Pharmakol. 202:594-596, 1943.

75. Günther, B. Toxicity of Benzedrine Sulfate in the White Mouse and in the Frog (Calyptocephalus Gayi). J. Pharmacol. exp. Ther. 76:375-377, 1942.

76. Frommel, E., et al. Pharmacological Study of Dextrorotatory and Levorotatory Pheneturide. Arch. int. Pharmacodyn. 122:15-31, 1959.

77. Chen, A. L. Preliminary Observations with Theophylline Mono-Ethanolamine. J. Pharmacol. exp. Ther. 45:1-5, 1932.

78. Garattini, S., et al. Antagonists of Reserpine Induced Eyelid Ptosis. Med. exp. (Basel) 3:252-259, 1960.

79. Wilson, S. P. and R. Tislow. Differential Antagonism of Reserpine Eyelid Closure by Imipramine and Amphetamine. Proc. Soc. exp. Biol. (N.Y.) 109:847-848, 1962.

80. Swinyard, E. A., et al. Studies on the Mechanism of Amphetamine Toxicity in Aggregated Mice. J. Pharmacol. exp. Ther. 132:97-102, 1961.

81. Ehrich, W. E. and K. B. Krumbhaar. The Effects of Large Doses of Benzedrine Sulphate on the Albino Rat: Functional and Tissue Changes. Ann. intern. Med. 10:1874-1888, 1957.

82. Smith, Kline and French Laboratories. Personal Communication.

83. Ehrich, W. E. et al. Experimental Studies upon the Toxicity of Benzedrine Sulphate in Various Animals. Amer. J. med. Sci. 198:785-803, 1939.

84. Searle, L. V. and C. W. Brown. Effect of Subcutaneous Injections of Benzedrine Sulfate on the Activity of White Rats. J. Exptl. Psychol. 22:480-490, 1938.

85. Garberg, L. and F. Sandberg. A Method for Quantitative Estimation of the Stimulant Effect of Analeptics on the Spontaneous Motility of Rats. Acta pharmacol. (Kbh.) 16:367-373, 1960.

86. Esser, A. Clinical, Anatomical and Spectrographic Investigations of the Central Nervous System in Acute Metal Poisoning with Particular Consideration of their Importance for Forensic Medicine and Industrial Pathology. Dtsch. Z. ges. gerichtl. Med. 25:239-317, 1935.

87. Munoz, C. and L. Goldstein. Influence of Adrenergic Blocking Drugs upon the EEG Analeptic Effect of dl-Amphetamine in Conscious Unrestrained Rabbits. J. Pharmacol. exp. Ther. 132:354-359, 1961.

88. Courvoisier, S. Pharmacodynamic Properties of the Chlorhydrate of Chloro-3 (Dimethyl-Amino-3' Propyl)-10 Phenothiazine (4.560 R.P.). Arch. int. Pharmacodyn. 92:305-361, 1953.

89. Cole, J. and P. Glees. Some Effects of Methyl-Phenidate (Ritalin) and Amphetamine on Normal and Neucotomized Monkeys. J. ment. Sci. 103:406-417, 1957.

90. Uyeda, A. and J. M. Fuster. The Effects of Amphetamine on Tachistoscopic Performance in the Monkey. Psychopharmacologia 3:463-467, 1962.

91. Hertting, G. et al. Effect of Drugs on the Uptake and Metabolism of H^3-Norepinephrine. J. Pharmacol. exp. Ther. 134:146-153, 1961.

92. Jaques, R. 5-Hydroxytryptamine Antagonists, with Special Reference to the Importance of Sympathomimetic Amines and Isopropyl-Noradrenaline. Helv. physiol. pharmacol. Acta. 14:269-278, 1956.

93. Ciba Pharmaceutical Company. Personal Communication.

94. Orahovats, P. D., et al. Pharmacology of Ethyl-1-(4-Aminophenethyl)-4-Phenylisonipecotate, Anileridine, a New Potent Synthetic Analgesic. J. Pharmacol. exp. Ther. 119:26-34, 1957.

95. Janssen, P. A. J., et al. Apomorphine-Antagonism in Rats. Arzneimittel-Forsch. 10:1003-1005, 1960.

96. Klee, P. and L. Laux. Further Investigations on Vomiting and the Action of Emetics. Deut. Arch. klin. Med. 149:189-208, 1925.

BIBLIOGRAPHY

97. Seiden, R. Veterinary Drugs in Current Use. Springer, New York, 1960.

98. Dandiya, P. C. and E. A. Sellers. Mechanism of the Hypnosis Prolongation Action of 5-Hydroxytryptamine and Some Sympathomimetic Amines. Arch. int. Pharmacodyn. 130:32-41, 1961.

99. Cook, L. et al. Epinephrine, Norepinephrine and Acetylcholine as Conditioned Stimuli for Avoidance Behavior. Science 131:990-991, 1960.

100. Chang, V. and M. J. Rand. Transmission Failure in Sympathetic Nerves Produced by Hemicholinium. Brit. J. Pharmacol. 15:588-600, 1960.

101. Cahen, R. L. and K. Tvede. Homatropine Methyl-Bromide: A Pharmacological Reëvaluation. J. Pharmacol. exp. Ther. 105:166-177, 1952.

102. Randall, L. O. and G. Lehmann. Pharmacological Studies on Analgesic Piperidine Derivatives. J. Pharmacol. exp. Ther. 93:314-328, 1948.

103. Schwartz, A. A Comparison of Two in vivo Methods Used for Assaying Anti-Ulcer Potency. Arch. int. Pharmacodyn. 127:203-210, 1960.

104. Willberg, M. A. Natural Resistance of Several Animals toward Atropine. Biochem. Z. 66:389-407, 1914.

105. Frommel, E. and C. Fleury. On the Paradoxical Mechanism of the Potentiation of the Soporific Effect of Barbiturates by Belladonna. Med. exp. (Basel) 3:257-263, 1960.

106. Domer, F. R. and F. M. Schueler. Investigations of the Amnesic Properties of Scopolamine and Related Compounds. Arch. int. Pharmacodyn. 127:449-458, 1960.

107. Ficklewirth, G. and A. Heffter. Resistance of the Rabbit to Atropine. Biochem. Z. 40:36-47, 1912.

108. White, R. P. and L. D. Boyajy. Neuropharmacological Comparison of Atropine, Scopolamine, Benactyzine, Diphenhydramine and Hydroxyzine. Arch. int. Pharmacodyn. 127:260-273, 1960.

109. Flury, F. and F. Zernik. Classification of Toxic and Lethal Doses for the Commonly Used Poisons and Research Animals. Abderhalden, Handbuch der biologischen Arbeitsmethoden. Abt. IV, Teil 7B:1289-1422, 1928.

110. Rice, W. B. and J. D. McColl. Antagonism of Psychotomimetic Agents in the Conscious Cat. Arch. int. Pharmacodyn. 127:249-259, 1960.

111. Abbott Laboratories. Personal Communication.

112. Loeb, C., et al. Electrophysiological Analysis of the Action of Atropine on the Central Nervous System. Rev. arch. ital. biol. 98:293-307, 1960.

113. Bainbridge, J. G. and D. M. Brown. Ganglion-Blocking Properties of Atropine-Like Drugs. Brit. J. Pharmacol. 15:147-151, 1960.

114. Paul-David, J., et al. Quantification of Effects of Depressant Drugs on EEG Activation Response. J. Pharmacol. exp. Ther. 129:69-74, 1960.

115. Usdin, E. and R. L. S. Amasi. Psychotropic and Related Compounds. Psychopharmacology Service Center Bulletin 2:17-93, 1963.

116. Brown, B. B. The Pharmacologic Activity of α-(4-Piperidyl)-Benzhydrol Hydrochloride (Azacyclonol Hydrochloride): An Ataractic Agent. J. Pharmacol. exp. Ther. 118:153-161, 1956.

117. Root, W. S. and F. G. Hofman. Physiological Pharmacology. Vol. 1: The Nervous System. Part A. Central Nervous System Drugs. Academic Press, New York and London, 1963.

118. Rümke, C. L. and J. Bout. The Influence of Previously Introduced Drugs on Hexobarbital Narcosis. Arch. exp. Path. Pharmakol. 240:218-223, 1960.

119. Tripod, J., et al. Experimental Differentiation of a Series of Central Nervous System Inhibitors. Arch. int. Pharmacodyn. 112:319-341, 1957.

120. Dhawan, B. N. and G. P. Gupta. Hypothermic and Antipyretic Activity of 4-Piperidyl Diphenyl Carbinol Hydrochloride (Azacyclonol). Arch. int. Pharmacodyn. 137:54-60, 1962.

121. Hahn, F. and A. Oberdorf. Comparative Investigations on the Antagonism of Bemegrid, Pentetrazol and Picrotoxin. Arch. int. Pharmacodyn. 135:9-30, 1962.

122. Gruber, C. M., et al. A Toxicological and Pharmacological Investigation of Sodium Sec-Butyl Ethyl Barbituric Acid (Butisol Sodium). J. Pharmacol. exp. Ther. 81:254-268, 1944.

123. MacFarlane, A. W. and J. S. McKenzie. The Pharmacology of a New Central Nervous System Stimulant, $\beta\beta$ Methyl Isopropyl Glutarimide. Arch. int. Pharmacodyn. 127:379-401, 1960.

124. Kuhn, W. L. and E. F. Von Maanen. Central Nervous System Effects of Thalidomide. J. Pharmacol. exp. Ther. 134:60-68, 1961.

125. Eddy, N. B. Studies of Morphine, Codeine and their Derivatives. IX. Methyl Ethers of the Morphine and Codeine Series. J. Pharmacol. exp. Ther. 55:127-135, 1935.

126. Underhill, F. P. and O. R. Johnson. A Comparative Study of New Ether Derivatives of Barbituric Acid. J. Pharmacol. exp. Ther. 35:441-448, 1929.

127. Lendle, L. Investigation on the Different Points of Attack of Some Narcotics in the Central Nervous System. Arch. exp. Path. Pharmakol. 143:108-116, 1929.

128. Jones, I. and E. V. Lynn. The Toxicity of Barbital Derivatives. J. Amer. pharm. Ass. 25:597-601, 1936.

129. Fitch, R. H. and E. E. McCandless. A Comparison of the Intraperitoneal and Oral Effects of the Barbituric Acid Derivatives. J. Pharmacol. exp. Ther. 42:266-267, 1931.

130. Elliott, K. A. C. and N. M. von Golder. The State of Factor I in Rat Brain: The Effects of Metabolic Conditions and Drugs. J. Physiol. (Lond.) 153:423-432, 1960

131. Schuster, R., et al. Pharmacological Data on the Analeptic Bemegride. Latvijas PSR Zinatnu Akad. 8:105-110, 1961.

132. Denisenko, P. P. The effect of Certain Esters of R, R'-Aminoethanol and Diphenylacetic Acid on the Central Nervous System. Farmakol. i Toksikol. 23:206-215, 1960.

133. Dobkin, A. B. Drugs Which Stimulate Affective Behavior. Anesthesia 15:273-279, 1961.

134. Oberdorf, A. and H. J. Meyer. On the Pharmacology of Megimid. Arch. exp. Path. Pharmak. 238:128-129, 1960.

135. Larsen, V. The General Pharmacology of Benzilic Acid Diethylaminoester Hydrochloride (Benactyzine NFN, Suavitil, Parasan). Acta pharmacol. (Kbh.) 11:405-420, 1955.

136. Farquharson, M. E. and R. G. Johnston. Antagonism of the Effects of Tremorine by Tropine Derivatives. Brit. J. Pharmacol. 14:559-566, 1960.

137. Boissier, J. R., et al. A New Simple Method for Exploring "Tranquilizing" Action: the Chimney Test. Med. Exptl. 3:81-84, 1960.

138. Bonta, I. L. New Application of the Motility Test in Screening Tranquilizing Drugs. Acta physiol. pharmacol. neerl. 7:519-522, 1958.

139. McColl, J. D. and W. B. Rice. Antagonism of Tremorine by Benactyzine and Dioxolane Analogs. Toxicol. appl. Pharmacol. 4:263-268, 1962.

140. Chen, G. The Anti-Tremorine Effect of Some Drugs as Determined by Haffner's Method of Testing Analgesia in Mice. J. Pharmacol. exp. Ther. 124:73-76, 1958.

141. Denisenko, P. P. Potentiation of Hypnotics and Anesthetics by Central Cholinolytics. Bull. Exp. Biol. Med. 49:593-597, 1960.

142. Frommel, E., et al. On the Differential Pharmacodynamics of Thymoanaleptics and Some "Neuroleptic" Substances in Animal Experimentation. Thérapie 15:1175-1198, 1960.

143. Navarro, M. G. Conditioned Emotional Responses and Psychotropic Drugs. Acta physiol. lat.-amer. 10:122-128, 1960.

144. Hanson, H. M. and D. A. Brodie. Use of the Restrained Rat Technique for Study of the Antiulcer Effect of Drugs. J. appl. Physiol. 15:291-294, 1960.

145. Sacra, P. et al. A Cat and Mouse Test for Studying Changes in Conflict Behavior. Canad. J. Biochem. 35:1151-1152, 1957.

146. Rose, C. L., et al. Toxicity of 3, 3'-Methylenebis (4-Hydroxycoumarin). Proc. Soc. exp. Biol. (N.Y.) 50:228-232, 1942.

147. Lupton, A. M. The Effect of Perfusion through the Isolated Liver on the Prothrombin Activity of Blood from Normal and Dicumarol Treated Rats. J. Pharmacol. exp. Ther. 89:306-312, 1947.

148. Boura, A. L. A. and A. F. Green. The Actions of Bretylium: Adrenergic Neurone Blocking and Other Effects. Brit. J. Pharmacol. 14:536-548, 1959.

149. Burroughs Wellcome & Co. (U. S. A.), Inc. Personal Communication.

150. Bhagat, B. and F. E. Shideman. Mechanism of the Positive Inotropic Responses to Bretylium and Guanethidine. Brit. J. Pharmacol. 20:56-62, 1963.

151. Green, A. F. and M. F. Sim. Diuresis in Rats: Effects of Sympathomimetic and Sympathetic Blocking Agents. Brit. J. Pharmacol. 17:237-242, 1960.

152. Ryd, G. Protective Effect of Bretylium on Noradrenaline Stores in Organs. Acta physiol. scand. 56:90-93, 1962.

153. Matsumoto, C. and A. Horita. Antagonism of Bretylium by Sumpathomimetic Amines. Nature 195:1212-1213, 1962.

154. Mantegazza, P., et al. The Peripheral Action of Hexamethonium and of Pentolinium. Brit. J. Pharmacol. 13:480-484, 1958.

155. Gessner, P. K. The Relationship between the Metabolic Fate and Pharmacological Action of Serotonin, Bufotenine and Psilocybin. J. Pharmacol. exp. Ther. 130:126-133, 1960.

156. Marczynski, T. and J. Vetulani. Further Investigations on the Pharmacological Properties of 5-Methoxy-N-Methyltryptamine. Diss. pharm. (Krakow) 12:67-84, 1960.

157. Monnier, M. and P. Krupp. Electrophysiological Action of Central Nervous System Stimulants. I. The Adrenergic, Cholinergic and Neurohumoral Serotonic Systems. Arch. int. Pharmacodyn. 127:337-360, 1960.

158. Bunag, R. D. and E. J. Walaszek. Differential Antagonism by RAS-Phenol of Responses to the Indolealkylamines. J. Pharmacol. exp. Ther. 136: 59-67, 1962.

159. Beck, R., et al. Stimulatory Effect of Psychotropic Drugs Demonstrated by Quantitative EEG. Pharmacologist 5:238, 1963.

160. Himwich, W. A. and E. Costa. Behavioral Changes Associated with Changes in Concentrations of Brain Serotonin. Fed. Proc. 19: 838-845, 1960.

161. Chen, B. M. and J. K. Weston. The Analgesic and Anesthetic Effect of 1-(1-Phenylcyclohexyl) Piperidine·HCl on the Monkeys. Anesth. Analg. Curr. Res. 39:132-137, 1960.

162. Molitor, H. The Use of Bulbocapnine in Pre-Anesthetic Medication. J. Pharmacol. exp. Ther. 56:85-96, 1936.

163. Grieg, M. E., et al. Bulbocapnine Catatonia in Mice. Fed. Proc. 17:373, 1958.

164. Zetler, G., et al. Pharmacological Properties of Antidepressive Drugs. Arch. exp. Path. Pharmakol. 238:486-501, 1960.

165. Glow, P. H. The Antagonism of Methyl Phenidate and Iproniazid to Bulbocapnine Catatonia in the Rat. Aust. J. exp. Biol. med. Sci. 40:499-504, 1962.

166. Farris, E. J. and J. Q. Griffith, Jr. The Rat in Laboratory Investigation. J. B. Lippincott Co., Philadelphia, 1949.

167. Walaszek, E. J. and J. E. Chapman. Bulbocapnine: An Adrenergic and Serotonin Blocking Agent. J. Pharmacol. exp. Ther. 137: 285-290, 1962.

168. Walaszek, E. J. and J. E. Chapman. Bulbocapnine: An Adrenergic and Serotonin Blocking Agent. Fed. Proc. 20:314, 1961.

169. Gantt, W. H. Cardiac Conditioning. Trans. 4th Res. Conf. Chemotherap. in Psychiat., Vet. Admin. 4:57-73, 1960.

170. Buchman, E. F. and C. P. Richter. Abolition of Bulbocapnine Catatonia by Cocaine. Arch. Neurol. Psychiat. (Chic.) 29:499, 1933.

171. Boura, A. and A. Green. Adrenergic Neurone Blockade and Other Acute Effects Caused by N-Benzyl-N'N"-Dimethylguanidine and its Ortho-Chloro Derivative. Brit. J. Pharmacol. 20:36-55, 1963.

172. Scott, C. C. and K. K. Chen. Comparison of the Action of 1-Ethyl Theobromine and Caffeine in Animals and Man. J. Pharmacol. exp. Ther. 82:89-97, 1944.

173. Funderburk, W. H., et al. EEG and Biochemical Findings with MAO Inhibitors. Ann. N. Y. Acad. Sci. 96:289-302, 1962.

174. Holm, T., et al. Pharmacology of a Series of Nuclear Substituted Phenyl-Tertiary-Butylamines with Particular Reference to Anorexi-

genic and Central Stimulating Properties. Acta Pharmacol. Toxicol. 17:121-136, 1960.

175. Akiyama, T. Studies on Whirling Syndromes Caused by Iminodipropionitrile. II. The Effect of Several Drugs on the Activity and Light Reaction of Circling Mice. Nippon Yakurigaku Zasshi 56:473-486, 1960.

176. Tripod, J., et al. Characterization of Central Effects of Serpasil (Reserpin, a New Alkaloid of Rauwolfia Serpentina B.) and of their Antagonistic Reactions. Arch. int. Pharmacodyn. 96:406-425, 1954.

177. Dews, P. B. The Measurement of the Influence of Drugs on Voluntary Activity in Mice. Brit. J. Pharmacol. 8:46, 1953.

178. Kreitmair, H. Antagonism between Barbiturates and Convulsants. Arch. exp. Path. Pharmakol. 187:607-616, 1937.

179. Nelson, F. New Apparatus for Experimental Methods Using Psychoactive Substances. Wiss. Z. Friedrich-Schiller-Univ. Jena, Math.-Naturwiss. Reihe 9:549-553, 1960.

180. Scott, C. C., et al. Further Study of Some 1-Substituted Theobromine Compounds. J. Pharmacol. exp. Ther. 86:113-119, 1946.

181. Verhave, T., et al. Effects of Various Drugs on Escape and Avoidance Behavior. Progr. Neurobiol. 3:267-279, 1958.

182. Salant, W. and J. B. Rieger. The Toxicity of Caffein. J. Pharmacol. exp. Ther. 1:572-574, 1910.

183. Sollmann, T. and J. B. Pilcher. The Actions of Caffein on the Mammalian Circulation. I. The Persistent Effects of Caffein on the Circulation. J. Pharmacol. exp. Ther. 3:19-92, 1911.

184. Schallek, W. and A. Kuehn. Effects of Drugs on Spontaneous and Activated EEG of Cat. Arch. int. Pharmacodyn. 120:319-333, 1959.

185. Malis, J. L., et al. Drug Effects on the Behavior of Self Stimulation in Monkeys. Fed. Proc. 19:23, 1960.

186. Cole, V. V., et al. The Toxicity of Strontium and Calcium. J. Pharmacol. exp. Ther. 71:1-5, 1941.

187. Ulrich, J. L. and V. A. Shternov. The Comparative Action of Hypertonic Solutions of the Chlorates and Chlorides of Potassium, Sodium, Calcium and Magnesium. J. Pharmacol. exp. Ther. 35:441-448, 1929.

188. Main, R. J. Mineral Salts as Factors in Urinary Prolan Concentrates. Endocrinology 24:523-525, 1939.

189. La Barre, J. Pharmacological Properties of Carbamyl-β-Methylcholine. I. Effects on Blood Pressure and Pancreas. Arch. int. Pharmacodyn. 106:245-259, 1956.

190. Kreitmair, H. A New Class of Cholinester. Arch. exp. Path. Pharmakol. 164:346-356, 1932.

191. O'Dell, T. B. Experimental Parameters in the Evaluation of Analgesics. Arch. int. Pharmacodyn. 134:154-174, 1961.

192. Frommel, E., et al. Analgesic Potency of Chlorpromazine in Comparison with Morphine and So-Called Morphinic Compounds. Helv. physiol. pharmacol. Acta 18:C24, 1960.

193. Castillo, J. del and T. E. Nelson, Jr. The Mode of Action of Carisoprodol. Ann. N. Y. Acad. Sci. 86:1960.

194. Franklin, K. J. The Pharmacology of Some Compounds Allied to Chloral and to Urethane. J. Pharmacol. exp. Ther. 42:1-7, 1931.

195. Führner, H. Contributions to Comparative Pharmacology. Arch. exp. Path. Pharmakol. 166:437-471, 1932.

196. Gros, O. and H. T. A. Haas. The Antagonism of Narcotics against Cardiazol. Arch. exp. Path. Pharmakol. 192:348-362, 1936.

197. Lehman, G. and P. K. Knoeffel. Trichlorethanol, Tribromethanol, Chloral Hydrate and Bromal Hydrate. J. Pharmacol. exp. Ther. 63:453-465, 1938.

198. Lewin, R. Scopolamine—Chloralhydrate Narcosis. Z. exp. Path. Ther. 18:61-66, 1916.

199. Lendle, L. A Contribution to the General Pharmacology of Narcosis: On the Narcotic Latitudes. Arch. exp. Path. Pharmakol. 132:214-245, 1928.

200. Wolf, A. and E. F. von Haxthausen. Toward the Analysis of the Effects of Some Centrally-Acting Sedative Substances. Arzneimittel-Forsch. 10:50-52, 1960.

201. Sollmann, T. A Comparative Study of the Dosage and Effects of Chloral Hydrate, Isopral and Bromural on Cats. J. Am. med. Assoc. 51:492, 1908.

202. Sigg, E. B. et al. The Influence of Some Nonbarbiturate Depressants on Central Polysynaptic Mechanisms. Arch. int. Pharmacodyn. 116:450-463, 1958.

203. Adams, W. D. The Comparative Toxicity of Chloral Alcoholate and Chloral Hydrate. J. Pharmacol. exp. Ther. 78:340-345, 1943.

204. Brown, B. B. CNS Drug Actions and Interaction in Mice. Arch. int. Pharmacodyn. 128: 391-414, 1960.

205. Dybing, O. and F. Dybing. Antagonism between Chloralose and Metrazole. Arch. exp. Path. Pharmakol. 199:435-437, 1942.

206. Heffter, A. Chloralglucose and its Action. Berl. klin. Wschr. 20:475, 1893.

207. Hanroit, M. M. and C. Richet. The Chloraloses. Arch. int. Pharmacodyn. 3:191-211, 1897.

208. Elliott, K. A. C. and F. Hobbigero. Gamma Aminobutyric Acid: Circulatory and Respiratory Effects in Different Species; Re-investigation of the Anti-Strychnine Action in Mice. J. Physiol. (Lond.) 146:70-84, 1959.

209. Daly, M. de B. and C. P. Luck. The Effects of Adrenaline and Noradrenalin on Pulmonary Haemodynamics with Special Reference to the Role of Reflexes from the Carotid Sinus Baroreceptors. J. Physiol. (Lond.) 145:108-123, 1959.

210. Hoffman-La Roche, Inc. Personal Communication.

211. Randall, L. O., et al. The Psychosedative Properties of Methaminodiazepoxide. J. Pharmacol. exp. Ther. 129:163-171, 1960.

212. Gershon, S. and W. J. Lang. A Psycho-Pharmacological Study of Some Indole Alkaloids. Arch. int. Pharmacodyn. 135:31-56, 1962.

213. Zbinder, G., et al. Experimental and Clinical Toxicology of Chlordiazepoxide (Librium). Toxicol. appl. Pharmacol. 3:619-637, 1961.

214. Stone, C. A., et al. Ganglionic Blocking Properties of 3-Methylamino-Isocomphane Hydrochloride (Mecamylamine); a Secondary Amine. J. Pharmacol. exp. Ther. 117:169-183, 1956.

215. Plummer, A. J., et al. Ganglionic Blockade by a New Bisquaternary Series Including Chlorisondamine Dimethochloride. J. Pharmacol. exp. Ther. 115:172-184, 1955.

216. Maxwell, R. A., et al. Factors Affecting the Blood Pressure Response of Mammals to the Ganglionic Blocking Agent, Chlorisondamine Chloride. J. Pharmacol. exp. Ther. 123:238-246, 1958.

217. Nickerson, M. and G. M. Nomaguchi. Adrenergic Blocking Action of Phenoxyethyl Analogues of Dibenzamine. J. Pharmacol. exp. Ther. 101:379-396, 1951.

218. Garattini, S. The Pressor Effect of Reserpine after Monoamine-Oxidase Inhibitors. Med. exp. (Basel) 2:252-259, 1960.

219. Raab, W. and R. J. Humphreys. Protective Effect of Adrenolytic Drugs Against Fatal Myocardial Epinephrine Concentrations. J. Pharmacol. exp. Ther. 88:268-276, 1946.

220. Harvey, S. C., et al. Blockade of Epinephrine-Induced Hyperglycemia. J. Pharmacol. exp. Ther. 104:363-376, 1952.

221. Labelle, A. and R. Tislow. Studies on Prophenpyridamine (Timeton) and Chlorprophenpyridamine (Chlortrimeton). J. Pharmacol. exp. Ther. 113:72-88, 1955.

222. Roth, F. E. and W. M. Govier. Comparative Pharmacology of Chlorpheniramine (Chlor-Trimeton) and its Optical Isomers. J. Pharmacol. exp. Ther. 124:347-349, 1958.

223. Schering Corporation. Personal Communication.

224. Hanson, H. M., et al. Drug Modification of Runway Behavior of Mice as Influenced by an Aversive Stimulus. Fed. Proc. 17:375, 1958.

225. Burton, R. M., et al. Interaction of Nicotinamide with Reserpine and Chlorpromazine. II. Some Effects on the Central Nervous System of the Mouse. Arch. int. Pharmacodyn. 128:253-259, 1960.

226. Fink, G. B. and E. Swinyard. Modification of Maximal Audiogenic and Electroshock Seizures in Mice by Psychopharmacologic Drugs. J. Pharmacol. exp. Ther. 127:318-324, 1959.

227. Boissier, J. R. Neuroleptics and Experimental Catatonia. Thérapie 15:73-77, 1960.

228. Irwin, S. Symposia on the Use of Tranquilizers in Veterinary Practice. Schering Corp., Bloomfield, N.J., 1958.

229. Weiss, B. and V. G. Laties. Effects of Amphetamine, Chlorpromazine and Pentobarbital on Behavioral Thermoregulation. J. Pharmacol. exp. Ther. 140:1-7, 1963.

230. Ito, S. The Effect of Several Tranquilizers on the Conditioned Avoidance Reaction of White Rats. Nippon Yakurigaku Zasshi 56: 377-386, 1960.

231. Ishikawa, S. A Pharmacological Study of Phenothiazine Derivatives. Nippon Yakurigaku Zasshi 56:498-513, 1960.

232. Jewett, R. and S. Norton. Drug Effects on Behavior of the Rat under Chronic Isolation. Pharmacologist 5:240, 1963.

233. Buchel, L. and J. Levy. Contribution to the Study of the Mechanism of Sedative Action of Reserpine. J. Physiol. (Paris) 52:727-733, 1960.

234. Yagi, K., et al. The Effect of Flavin Adenine Dinucleotide on the Electroencephalogram Modified by Chlorpromazine. J. Neurochem. 5:304-306, 1960.

235. Domenjoz, R. and W. Theobald. The Pharmacology of Tofranil (N-(3-Dimethyl-aminopropyl)-Iminodibenzylhydrochloride). Arch. int. Pharmacodyn. 120:450-489, 1959.

236. Komendantova, M. V. The Meaning of the Ion Component in the Pharmacodynamics of Aminazine. Farmakol. i Toksikol. 23:99-105, 1960.

237. Enge, S. and H. Lechner. An Experimental Contribution to the Mode of Drug Action in Animals. Wien. Z. Nervenheilk. u. Grenzg. 17:309-323, 1960.

238. Barkov, N. K. Analgetic Properties of Phenothiazine Derivatives. Farmakol. i Toksikol. 23:311-315, 1960.

239. Adey, W. R. and C. W. Dunlop. Amygdaloid and Peripheral Influences on Caudate and Pallidal Units in the Cat and Effects of Chlorpromazine. Exp. Neurol. 2:348-363, 1960.

240. Kaada, B. R. and H. Bruland. Blocking of the Cortically Induced Behavioral Attention (Orienting) Response by Chlorpromazine. Psychopharmacologia 1:372-388, 1960.

241. Feldman, S. and M. Eliakim. Observations on the Mechanism of Blood Pressure Changes Following Chlorpromazine Administration in the Cat. Arch. int. Pharmacodyn. 141:340-356, 1958.

242. Leutova, F. A. The Problem of the Mechanism of the Action of Aminazine and Physical Cooling on the Therapeutic Reflexes. Zh. Nevropat. Psikhiat. 60:210-219, 1960.

243. Polezhayev, E. F. Action of Aminazine and Adrenaline in Small Doses on the Formation of Cortical Coordination. Zh. Nevropat. Psikhiat. 60:568-576, 1960.

244. Agangants, E. K. Effects of Chlorpromazine and Ethylene on Conditioned Reflexes in Dogs. Pavlov J. higher nerv. Activ. 10:899-908, 1960.

245. Khananashbili, M. M. The Mechanism of Action of Chlorpromazine on Higher Nervous Activity. Farmakol. i Toksikol. 23:295-299, 1960.

246. Fuller, J. L., et al. Effects of Chlorpromazine upon Psychological Development in the Puppy. Psychopharmacologia 1:393-407, 1960.

247. Domino, E. F. and S. Ueki. An Analysis of the Electrical Burst Phenomenon in Some Rhinencephalic Structures of the Dog and Monkey. Electroenceph. clin. Neurophysiol. 12:635-648, 1960.

248. Weitzman, E. and G. Ross. Behavioral Method for Study of Pain Perception in Monkeys. Neurology (Minneap.) 12:264-272, 1962.

249. Browning, H. C., et al. Weights of Thymus and Seminal Vesicle in Castrate Mice as Altered by Intraperitoneal and Subcutaneous Injections of Testerone. Tox. Rep. Biol. Med. 19:753-760, 1961.

250. Stone, G. C., et al. Behavioral and Pharmacological Studies of Thiopropazate, a Potent Tranquilizing Agent. Arch. int. Pharmacodyn. 127:85-103, 1960.

251. Chen, G. and B. Bohner. A Study of Certain CNS Depressants. Arch. int. Pharmacodyn. 125:1-20, 1960.

252. Tanaka, K. and Y. Kawasaki. A Group of

Compounds Possessing Anticonvulsant Activity in the Maximal Electroshock Seizure Test. Jap. J. Pharmacol. 6:115-121, 1957.

253. Luduena, F. P., et al. Effect of Adrenergic Blockers and Related Compounds on the Toxicity of Epinephrine in Rats. Arch. int. Pharmacodyn. 122:111-122, 1959.

254. Busch, V. G., et al. Electrophysiological Analysis of the Action of Hemoleptic and Tranquilizing Substances (Phenothiazine, Meprobamate) on the Spinal Motor System. Arzneimittel-Forsch. 10:217-223, 1960.

255. Piala, J. J., et al. Pharmacology of Benzhydroflumethazide (Naturetin). J. Pharmacol. exp. Ther. 134:273-280, 1961.

256. Bacharach, A. L. The Effect of Ingested Vitamin E (Tocopherol) on Vitamin A Storage in the Liver of the Albino Rat. Quart. J. Pharm. 14:138-149, 1940.

257. Fromherz, K. Larocain, a New Local Anesthetic. Arch. exp. Path. Pharmakol. 158:368-380, 1930.

258. Hooper, C. W. and E. Becker. A Quantitative Comparison of Toxicity of Alkamine Esters of Aromatic Acids Used as Local Anesthetics. Am. J. Physiol. 68:120, 1924.

259. Rose, C. L., et al. Studies in the Pharmacology of Local Anesthetics. III. Comparison of Gamma-(2-Methyl Piperidine) Propyl Benzoate Hydrochloride with Cocaine and Procaine on Experimental Animals. J. Lab. clin. Med. 15:731-735, 1930.

260. Eicholtz, F. and C. Hoppe. The Convulsive Action of Local Anesthetics and the Effect of Mineral Salts and Adrenaline. Arch. exp. Path. Pharmakol. 173:687-696, 1933.

261. Brodie, B. B. Comparison of Central Actions of Cocaine and LSD. Fed. Proc. 16: 284, 1957.

262. Bogdanski, D. and S. Spector. Comparison of Central Actions of Cocaine and LSD. Fed. Proc. 16:284, 1957.

263. Wingard, C. and R. S. Teague. Potentiation of the Pressor Response to Epinephrine and Sympathomimetic Aldehydes. Arch. int. Pharmacodyn. 116:54-64, 1958.

264. Chen, G. and B. Bohner. The Anti-Reserpine Effects of Certain Centrally-Acting Agents.

J. Pharmacol. exp. Ther. 131:179-184, 1961.

265. MacMillan, W. H. A Hypothesis Concerning the Effect of Cocaine on the Action of Sympathomimetic Amines. Brit. J. Pharmacol. 14:385-391, 1959.

266. Gurd, M. R. The Physiological Action of Dihydroxyphenylethylamine and Sympatol. Quart. J. and Year Book of Pharm. 10:188-211, 1937.

267. Kissel, J. W., et al. The Pharmacology of Prodilidine Hydrochloride, a New Analgetic Agent. J. Pharmacol. exp. Ther. 134:332-340, 1961.

268. Poe, C. F. and J. G. Strong. The Toxicity of Certain Compounds for Male and Female Rats of Different Ages. J. Pharmacol. exp. Ther. 58:239-242, 1936.

269. Ercoli, N. and M. N. Lewis. Studies on Analgesics. J. Pharmacol. exp. Ther. 84: 301-317, 1945.

270. Eddy, N. B. and M. Sumwalt. Studies of Morphine, Codeine and their Derivatives. XV. 2,4-Dinitrophenylmorphine. J. Pharmacol. exp. Ther. 67:127-141, 1939.

271. O'Dell, T. B., et al. Pharmacology of a Series of New 2-Substituted Pyridine Derivatives with Emphasis on their Analgesic and Interneuronal Blocking Properties. J. Pharmacol. exp. Ther. 128:65-74, 1960.

272. Goldberg, B., et al. Colchicine Derivatives. I. Toxicity in Mice and Effects on Mouse Sarcoma 180. Cancer 3:124-129, 1950.

273. Streicher, E. Toxicity of Colchicine, Di-Isopropyl Fluorophosphate, Intocostrin, and Potassium Cyanide in Mice at 4°C. Proc. Soc. exp. Biol. (N.Y.) 76:536-538, 1951.

274. Sollmann, T. A Manual of Pharmacology and its Application to Therapeutics and Toxicology. W. B. Saunders Co. (7th ed.), Philadelphia, 1948.

275. Ferguson, F. C., Jr. Colchicine. I. General Pharmacology. J. Pharmacol. exp. Ther. 106: 261-270, 1952.

276. Santav, F., et al. Mitolytic Action and Toxicity of New Substances Isolated from Colchicine. Arch. int. Pharmacodyn. 84:257-268, 1950.

BIBLIOGRAPHY

277. Maurel, M. Influence of Route of Adminis-
tration on the Production of Colchicine-
Diarrhea in the Rabbit. C. R. Soc. Biol.
(Paris) 67:768-769, 1909.

278. Dixon, W. E. and W. Malden. Colchicine
with Special Reference to its Mode of Action
and Effect on Bone Marrow. J. Physiol.
(Lond.) 37:50-76, 1908.

279. Fernandez, E. and A. Cerletti. Studies on
the Hypotensive Mechanism of Protoveratrine.
Arch. int. Pharmacodyn. 100:425-435, 1955.

280. Castillo, J. C. and E. J. de Beer. The
Neuromuscular Blocking Action of Succinyl-
choline (Diacetylcholine). J. Pharmacol. exp.
Ther. 99:458-464, 1950.

281. Bovet, D., et al. Studies on Synthetic
Curare-Like Poisons. Arch. int. Pharmacodyn.
88:1-50, 1951.

282. Walton, R. P., et al. Inotropic Activity of
Catechol Isomers and a Series of Related
Compounds. J. Pharmacol. exp. Ther. 125:
202-207, 1959.

283. Paton, W. D. M. and E. J. Zamis. Clinical
Potentialities of Certain Bisquaternary Salts
Causing Neuromuscular and Ganglionic Block.
Nature (Lond.) 162:810, 1948.

284. Setniker, I., et al. Amino-Methylchromes,
Brain Stem Stimulants and Pentobarbital
Antagonists. J. Pharmacol. exp. Ther. 128:
176-181, 1960.

285. Day, M. and M. Rand. Evidence for a Competitive Antagonism of Guanethidine by Dex-
amphetamine. Brit. J. Pharmacol. 20:17-28,
1963.

286. Buchel, L., et al. A Contribution to the
Study of the Effects of Hydrazine-2-Phenyl-
3-Propane (PIH) on the Central Nervous System, Compared with Those of 1-Isonicotinyl-
2-Isopropylhydrazide (Iproniazid). IV. Influence on Analgesia Induced by 1-Methadone.
Agressologie 1:389-396, 1960.

287. Hamilton, C. L. Effects of LSD-25 and
Amphetamine on a Running Response in the
Rat. Arch. gen. Psychiat. 2:104-109, 1960.

288. Sergio, C. Effects of Bulbocapnine in Some
Decorticated Rabbits. Riv. Neurobiol. 6:51-
53, 1960.

289. Jarvik, M. E. and S. Chorover. Impairment

by Lysergic Acid Diethylamide of Accuracy
in Performance of a Delayed Alternation
Test in Monkeys. Psychopharmacologia 1:
221-230, 1960.

290. Kleindorf, G. B. and J. T. Halsey. A Study
of the Relative Efficiency as "Basal Anesthetics" of Avertin, Amytal, Chloral, Dial,
and Isopropyl Allyl Barbituric Acid. J. Pharmacol. exp. Ther. 43:449-456, 1931.

291. Peterson, I. and E. Bohm. Differences in
Sensitivity to Dial of Motor Effects Elicited
by Stimulation of Fore- and Hindlimb Areas
of the Cat's Motor Cortex. Acta physiol.
scand. 29:143-146, 1953.

292. Schneider, J. A. and F. F. Yonkman. Action
of Serotonin (5-Hydroxytryptamine) on Vagal
Afferent Impulses in the Cat. Am. J. Physiol.
174:127-134, 1953.

293. O'Leary, J. F. Cardiovascular Actions of
1, 4-Bis (1, 4-Benzodioxan-2-yl-Methyl) Piperazine (McN-181, Dibozane), a New Adrenergic
Blocking Agent. Fed. Proc. 12:355, 1953.

294. Yelnosky, L. and L. C. Mortimer. A Brief
Study of the Sympathomimetic Cardiovascular
Effects of Bretylium. Arch. int. Pharmacodyn.
130:200-206, 1961.

295. Rapela, C. E. and H. D. Green. Adrenergic
Blockade by Dibozane. J. Pharmacol. exp.
Ther. 132:29-41, 1961.

296. Powell, C. E. and I. H. Slater. Blocking of
Inhibitory Adrenergic Receptors by a Dichloro
Analog of Isoproterenol. J. Pharmacol. exp.
Ther. 122:480-488, 1958.

297. Eli Lilly and Company. Personal Communication.

298. Goldstein, L. and C. Munoz. Influence of
Adrenergic Stimulant and Blocking Drugs on
Cerebral Electrical Activity in Curarized
Animals. J. Pharmacol. exp. Ther. 132:345-
353, 1961.

299. Levy, B. Adrenergic Blockade Produced by
the Dichloro Analogs of Epinephrine, Arterenol
and Isoproterenol. J. Pharmacol. exp. Ther.
127:150-156, 1959.

300. Ahlquist, R. P. and B. Levy. Adrenergic
Receptive Mechanism of Canine Ileum. J.
Pharmacol. exp. Ther. 127:146-149, 1959.

301. Hall, W. J. The Action of Tyramine on the

Dog Isolated Atrium. Brit. J. Pharmacol. 20: 245-253, 1963.

302. Fleming, W. W. and D. F. Hawkins. The Actions of Dichloroisoproternol in the Dog Heart-Lung Preparation and Isolated Guinea Pig Atrium. J. Pharmacol. exp. Ther. 129: 1-10, 1960.

303. Lendle, L. Digitalis Substances and Related Glycosides Working on the Heart (Digitaloids). Heffter's Hdb. E. 1:11-265, 1935.

304. Röthlin, E. On the Pharmacology of the Hydrated Natural Mother Seed Alkaloids. Helv. physiol. pharmacol. Acta 2:C48, 1944.

305. Naranjo, P. and E. B. de Naranjo. Pressor Effect of Histamine in the Rabbit. J. Pharmacol. exp. Ther. 123:16-21, 1958.

306. West, T. C. and J. M. Dille. Reversal of Depressor Effect of TEA. J. Pharmacol. exp. Ther. 108:233-239, 1953.

307. Buchwald, M. E. and G. S. Eadie. The Toxicology of Dilaudid Injected Intravenously into Mice. J. Pharmacol. exp. Ther. 71:197-202, 1941.

308. Eddy, N. B. and J. G. Reid. Studies of Morphine, Codeine and their Derivatives. VII. Dihydromorphine (Paramorphan), Dihydromorphinone (Dilaudid), and Dihydrocodeinone (Dicodide). J. Pharmacol. exp. Ther. 52: 468-493, 1934.

309. Friebel, H. and C. Reichle. Analgesia and Analgesia-Enhancing Effects of Chlorpromazine. Arch. exp. Path. Pharmakol. 226:551-573, 1955.

310. Eddy, N. B. and H. A. Howes. Studies of Morphine, Codeine and their Derivatives. J. Pharmacol. exp. Ther. 53:430-439, 1935.

311. Horton, R. G., et al. The Acute Toxicity of Di-Isopropyl Fluorophosphate. J. Pharmacol. exp. Ther. 87:414-429, 1946.

312. Koelle, G. B. and A. Gilman. The Relationship between Cholinesterase Inhibition and the Pharmacological Action of Di-Isopropyl Fluorophosphate (DFP). J. Pharmacol. exp. Ther. 87:421-434, 1946.

313. Cook, D. L., et al. Pharmacology of a New Autonomic Ganglion Blocking Agent, 2,6-Dimethyl-1,1-Diethyl Piperidinium Bromide (SC-1950). J. Pharmacol. exp. Ther. 99:435-443, 1950.

314. Chen, G., et al. Pharmacology of 1,1-Dimethyl-4-Phenylpiperazinium Iodide, A Ganglionic Stimulating Agent. J. Pharmacol. exp. Ther. 103:330-336, 1951.

315. Tainter, M. L. and W. C. Cutting. Miscellaneous Actions of Dinitrophenol. Repeated Administrations, Antidotes, Fatal Doses, Antiseptic Tests and Actions of Some Isomers. J. Pharmacol. exp. Ther. 49:187-208, 1933.

316. Spencer, H. C., et al. Toxicological Studies on Laboratory Animals of Certain Alkyldinitrophenols Used in Agriculture. J. industr. Hyg. 30:10-25, 1948.

317. Tainter, M. L., et al. Metabolic Activity of Compounds Related to Dinitrophenol. J. Pharmacol. exp. Ther. 53:58-66, 1935.

318. Magne, H., et al. Pharmacodynamic Action of the Nitrated Phenols: An Agent Increasing Cellular Oxidations, 2,4-Dinitrophenol. Ann. physiol. physiochim. biol. 8:1-50, 1932.

319. Tainter, M. L. and W. C. Cutting. Febrile, Respiratory and Some Other Actions of Dinitrophenol. J. Pharmacol. exp. Ther. 48: 410-429, 1933.

320. Way, E. L. and W. C. Herbert. The Effect of Sodium Pentobarbital on the Toxicity of Certain Antihistamines. J. Pharmacol. exp. Ther. 104:115-121, 1952.

321. Gruhzit, O. M. and R. A. Fisken. A Toxicological Study of Two Histamine Antagonists of the Benzhydryl Alkamine Ether Group. J. Pharmacol. exp. Ther. 89:227-233, 1947.

322. De Salva, S. and R. Evans. Anticonvulsive Character of Styramate and Other Depressant Drugs. Toxicol. appl. Pharmacol. 2:397-402, 1960.

323. Chen, G. and B. Bohner. A Study of Central Nervous System Stimulants. J. Pharmacol. exp. Ther. 123:212-215, 1958.

324. Loew, E. R. Pharmacology of Antihistamine Compounds. Physiol. Rev. 27:542-573, 1947.

325. Sachs, B. A. The Toxicity of Benadryl: Report of a Case and Review of the Literature. Ann. intern. Med. 29:135-144, 1948.

326. De Salva, S. and R. Evans. Continuous Intravenous Infusion of Strychnine in Rats: II. Antagonism by Various Drugs. Arch. int. Pharmacodyn. 125:355-361, 1960.

327. Blaschko, H. and T. L. Chrusciel. The Decarboxylation of Amino Acids Related to Tyrosine and their Awakening Action in Reserpine-Treated Mice. J. Physiol. (Lond.) 151:272-284, 1960.

328. Page, I. H. and R. Reed. Hypertensive Effect of L-Dopa and Related Compounds in the Rat. Am. J. Physiol. 143:122-125, 1945.

329. Kato, R. Effects of Pre-Electroshock Treatment on the Duration of Tranquilizer Effect, and on the Contents of Brain Serotonin. Nippon Yakurigaku Zasshi 56:1046-1053, 1960.

330. Burn, J. H. and M. J. Rand. The Depressor Action of Dopamine and Adrenaline. Brit. J. Pharmacol. 13:471-479, 1958.

331. Costa, E., et al. Brain Concentration of Biogenic Amines and EEG Patterns of Rabbits. J. Pharmacol. exp. Ther. 130:81-88, 1960.

332. Rowe, L. W. The Comparative Pharmacologic Action of Ephedrine and Adrenalin. J. Am. pharm. Ass. 16:912-918, 1927.

333. Chen, K. K. and C. F. Schmidt. The Action and Clinical Use of Ephedrine. J. Amer. med. Ass. 87:836-842, 1926.

334. Chen, K. K. The Acute Toxicity of Ephedrine. J. Pharmacol. exp. Ther. 27:61-76, 1926.

335. Hauschild, F. On the Pharmacology of 1-Phenyl-2-Methylaminopropane (Pervitin). Arch. exp. Path. Pharm. 191:465-481, 1939.

336. Watson, R. H. J. Constitutional Differences between Two Strains of Rats with Different Behavioral Characteristics. Advanc. Psychosomatic Med. 1:160-165, 1960.

337. Grishina, V. M. Antihypnotic Action of Ephedrine. Farmakol. i Toksikol. 23:287-295, 1960.

338. Axelrod, J. and R. Tomchick. Increased Rate of Metabolism of Epinephrine and Norepinephrine by Sympathomimetic Amines. J. Pharmacol. exp. Ther. 130:367-369, 1960.

339. Burn, J. H. and M. J. Rand. The Action of Sympathetic Amines in Animals Treated with Reserpine. J. Physiol. (Lond.) 144:314-336, 1958.

340. Lands, A. M., et al. The Pharmacology of

341. Bovet, D. and G. Bovet-Nitti. Medications of the Autonomic Nervous System. S. Karger, New York, 1948.

342. Levy, J. and E. Michel-Ber. A Hypothesis about the Mechanisms of Action of Monamine Oxidase Inhibitors at the Central Nervous System Level. C. R. Acad. Sci. (Paris) 250: 415-417, 1960.

343. Raab, W. and R. J. Humphreys. Protective Effect of Adrenolytic Drugs against Fatal Myocardial Epinephrine Concentrations. J. Pharmacol. exp. Ther. 88:268-276, 1946.

344. Smythies, J. R. and C. K. Levy. The Comparative Pharmacology of Some Mescaline Analogues. J. ment. Sci. 106;531-536, 1960.

345. Savoldi, F., et al. Action of a Water-Soluble Derivative of Theobromine on the Cerebral Circulation and Cortical Electrical Activity of the Rabbit. Arch. ital. Sci. farmacol. 10: 231-240, 1960.

346. Spector, W. S. Handbook of Toxicology. Vol. I. WADC Technical Report 55-16, 1955.

347. Kostos, V. J. and J. J. Kocsis. Tissue Serotonin (5-HT) Levels in Colchicine Treated Rats and Rabbits. Pharmacologist 5:247, 1963.

348. Röthlin, E. Investigation of Ergotamine, a Specific Alkaloid of Ergot. Arch. int. Pharmacodyn. 27:459-479, 1923.

349. Röthlin, E. The Pharmacological Properties of a New Alkaloid of Ergot, Ergobasine. C. R. Soc. Biol. (Paris) 119:1302-1304, 1935.

350. Laurence, D. R. and R. S. Stacey. Mechanism of the Prevention of Nicotine Convulsions by Hexamethonium and by Adrenaline Blocking Agents. Brit. J. Pharmacol. 8:62-65, 1953.

351. Barger, G. The Alkaloids of Ergot. Heffter's Hdb. E. 6:84-222, 1938.

352. Sandoz Pharmaceuticals. Personal Communication.

353. Ginzel, K. H. The Effect of d-Lysergic Acid Diethylamide and Other Drugs on the Carotid Sinus Reflex. Brit. J. Pharmacol. 13:250-259, 1958.

354. Mayer, S., et al. The Effect of Adrenergic

N-Alkyl Homologues of Epinephrine. J. Pharmacol. exp. Ther. 90:110-119, 1947.

Blocking Agents on Some Metabolic Actions of Catecholamines. J. Pharmacol. exp. Ther. 134:18-27, 1961.

355. Graham, G., et al. Influence of Fluoroacetate on Renal Acid Secretion. Fed. Proc. 12:325, 1953.

356. Furchgott, R. F. The Effect of Sodium Fluoroacetate on the Contractility and Metabolism of Intestinal Smooth Muscle. J. Pharmacol. exp. Ther. 99:1-15, 1950.

357. Matthews, R. J. and B. J. Roberts. The Effect of Gamma-Aminobutyric Acid on Synaptic Transmission in Autonomic Ganglia. J. Pharmacol. exp. Ther. 132:19-22, 1961.

358. Rech, R. H. and E. F. Domino. Effects of Gamma-Aminobutyric Acid on Chemically and Electrically Evoked Activity in the Isolated Cerebral Cortex of the Dog. J. Pharmacol. exp. Ther. 130:59-67, 1960.

359. Gulati, O. D. and H. C. Stanton. Some Effects on the Central Nervous System of Gamma-Amino-n-Butyric Acid (GABA) and Certain Related Amino Acids Administered Systemically and Intracerebrally to Mice. J. Pharmacol. exp. Ther. 129:175-185, 1960.

360. Winter, C. A. and J. T. Lehman. Studies on Synthetic Curarizing Agents. J. Pharmacol. exp. Ther. 100:489-501, 1950.

361. Bovet, D., et al. Studies on Synthetic Curare-Like Poisons. Arch. int. Pharmacodyn. 80:172-188, 1949.

362. Longo, V. G. Effects of Scopolamine and Atropine on Electroencephalographic and Behavioral Reactions Due to Hypothalamic Stimulation. J. Pharmacol. exp. Ther. 116:198-208, 1956.

363. Maxwell, R. A., et al. Pharmacology of (2(Octahydro-1-Azocinyl)-Ethyl)-Guanidine Sulfate (SU-5864). J. Pharmacol. exp. Ther. 128:22-29, 1960.

364. Bogaert, M., et al. On the Pharmacology of Guanethidine. Arch. int. Pharmacodyn. 134:224-236, 1961.

365. Cass, R. and T. Spriggs. Tissue Amine Levels and Sympathetic Blockade after Guanethidine and Bretylium. Brit. J. Pharmacol. 17:442-450, 1961.

366. Cass, R., et al. Norepinephrine Depletion

as a Possible Mechanism of Action of Guanethidine (SU-5864), a New Hypotensive Agent. Proc. Soc. exp. Biol. (N.Y.) 103:871-872, 1960.

367. Dagirmanjian, R. The Effects of Guanethidine on the Noradrenaline Content of the Hypothalamus in the Cat and Rat. J. Pharm. Pharmacol. 15:518-521, 1963.

368. Gunn, J. A. The Pharmacological Action of Harmaline. Trans. Roy. Soc. Edin. 47:245-272, 1909.

369. Ahmed, A. and N. R. W. Taylor. The Analysis of Drug-Induced Tremor in Mice. Brit. J. Pharmacol. 14:350-354, 1959.

370. Pellmont, B. and F. A. Steiner. Influence on a Conditioned Reflex by Drugs with Effects on Monamine Metabolism in the Central Nervous System. Psychiat. et Neurol. (Basel) 140:216-219, 1960.

371. Spector, S., et al. Evidence for Release of Brain Amines by Reserpine in Presence of Monoamine Oxidase Inhibitors: Implication of Monoamine Oxidase in Norepinephrine Metabolism in Brain. J. Pharmacol. exp. Ther. 130:256-261, 1960.

372. Goldberg, L. I. and A. Sjoerdsma. Effects of Several Monoamine Oxidase Inhibitors on the Cardiovascular Actions of Naturally Occurring Amines in the Dog. J. Pharmacol. exp. Ther. 127:212-218, 1959.

373. Hara, S. and I. Mori. Investigation of Poisons of the Extrapyramidal Paths. II. Pharmacological Contribution to Harmin. Jap. J. Med. Sc. IV Pharm. 7:78-79, 1933.

374. Gunn, J. A. and R. C. MacKeith. The Pharmacological Actions of Harmol. Quart. J. Pharm. 4:33-51, 1931.

375. Lewin, L. Chemistry and Pharmacological Action of Banisteria Caapi Spr. Arch. exp. Path. Pharmakol. 129:133-149, 1928.

376. Goldberg, L. I. and F. M. DeCosta. Selective Depression of Sympathetic Transmission by Intravenous Administration of Iproniazid and Harmine. Proc. Soc. exp. Biol. (N.Y.) 105:223-227, 1960.

377. Marshall, F. N. and J. P. Long. Pharmacologic Studies on Some Compounds Structurally Related to the Hemicholinium HC-3. J. Pharmacol. exp. Ther. 127:236-240, 1959.

378. Kase, Y. and H. L. Borison. Central Respiratory Depressant Effect of "Hemicholinium." Fed. Proc. 16:311, 1957.

379. Zablocka, B. and D. Esplin. Evidence for a Cholinergic Link in "Direct" Spinal Inhibition. Pharmacologist 5:237, 1963.

380. Seifter, J. and A. J. Begany. Studies on the Action of a Synthetic Heparinoid. Am. J. med. Sci. 216:234-235, 1948.

381. Montague, D., et al. Bradykinin: Vascular Relaxant, Cardiac Stimulant. Science 141: 907-908, 1963.

382. Wenke, M. Relation between the Heparin Dose and the Esterolytic Activity Level in the Blood Serum of Rats. Arch. int. Pharmacodyn. 134:417-425, 1961.

383. Gillis, C. N. and C. W. Nash. The Initial Pressor Actions of Bretylium Tosylate and Guanethidine Sulfate and their Relation to Release of Catecholamines. J. Pharmacol. exp. Ther. 134:1-7, 1961.

384. Wolff, R. and J. J. Brignon. A Study of the Serum-Clearing Activity of Several Heparin-Like Substances in vitro. Arch. int. Pharmacodyn. 121:255-267, 1959.

385. Davey, M. J., et al. The Effects of Nialamide on Adrenergic Functions. Brit. J. Pharmacol. 20:121-134, 1963.

386. Salmoiraghi, G. C., et al. Effects of d-Lysergic Acid Diethylamine and its Brom Derivative on Cardiovascular Responses to Serotonin and on Arterial Pressure. J. Pharmacol. exp. Ther. 119:240-247, 1957.

387. Grollman, A. The Effect of Various Hypotensive Agents on the Arterial Blood Pressure of Hypertensive Rats and Dogs. J. Pharmacol. exp. Ther. 14:263-270, 1955.

388. Della Bella, D. and F. Rognoni. Neurovegetative Control of Gastric Motility in the Isolated Nerve-Stomach Preparation of the Rat. J. Pharmacol. exp. Ther. 134:184-189, 1961.

389. Kennedy, W. P. Sodium Salt of C-C-Cyclohexenylmethyl-N-Methyl Barbituric Acid (Evipan) Anaesthesia in Laboratory Animals. J. Pharmacol. exp. Ther. 50:347-353, 1934.

390. Buller, R. H., et al. The Potentiating Effect of 4,5-Dihydro-6-Methyl-2[2-(4-Pyridyl)-Ethyl]-3-Pyridazinone (U-320) on Hexobarbital Hypnosis. J. Pharmacol. exp. Ther. 134:95-99, 1961.

391. Reinhard, J. F., et al. Pharmacologic Characteristics of 1-(Ortho-Toluoxy)-2,3-Bis-(2,2,2-Trichloro-1 Hydroxyethoxy)-Propane. J. Pharmacol. exp. Ther. 106:444-452, 1952.

392. Bush, M. T., et al. The Metabolic Fate of Evipal (Hexobarbital) and of "Nor-Evipal." J. Pharmacol. exp. Ther. 108:104-111 (1953).

393. Maloney, A. H. and R. Hertz. Sodium N-Methyl-Cyclohexenyl-Methyl-Barbituric Acid (Evipal): Hypnosis, Anesthesia and Toxicity. J. Pharmacol. exp. Ther. 54:77-83, 1935.

394. Werner, H. W., et al. A Comparative Study of Several Ultrashortacting Barbiturates, Nembutal, and Tribromethanol. J. Pharmacol. exp. Ther. 60:189-197, 1937.

395. Shimamoto, K., et al. Peripheral Action of the Ganglion Blocking Agents. Jap. J. Pharmacol. 5:66-76, 1955.

396. Takagi, H. and T. Ban. Effect of Psychotropic Drugs on the Limbic System of the Cat. Jap. J. Pharmacol. 10:7-14, 1960.

397. Lin, T. M., et al. 3-β-Aminoethyl-1,2,4-Triazole, a Potent Stimulant of Gastric Secretion. J. Pharmacol. exp. Ther. 134:88-94, 1961.

398. Lands, A. M., et al. The Pharmacological Properties of Three New Antihistaminic Drugs. J. Pharmacol. exp. Ther. 95:45-52, 1949.

399. Schmidt, G. W. and A. Stähelin. Histamine Sensitivity and Anaphylaxis Reaction. Z. Innunitatstorsch. 60:222-238, 1929.

400. Parrot, J. L., et al. Acute Intoxication of the Cobaye through Gastric Administration of Histamine Alone or Associated with Putrescence. 17th Int. Physiol. Cong., 1947: p. 378.

401. Camus, L. Hordenine, the Degree of the Toxic Symptoms of Intoxication. C. R. Acad. Sci. (Paris) 142:110-113, 1906.

402. Barger, G. and H. H. Dale. Chemical Structure and Sympathomimetic Action of Amines. J. Physiol. (Lond.) 41:19-59, 1910.

403. Craver, N. The Activities of 1-Hydrazinophthalazine (Ba-5968), a Hypotensive Agent.

J. Amer. pharm. Ass., sci. Ed. 40:559-564, 1961.

404. Schmitt, H. Adrenolytic, Noradrenolytic and Sympatholytic Action of Dibenzyline (SKF 688A). Arch. int. Pharmacodyn. 109:263-270, 1957.

405. Rocha e Silva, M., et al. Potentiation of Duration of the Vasodilator Effect of Bradykinin by Sympatholytic Drugs and Reserpine. J. Pharmacol. exp. Ther. 128:217-226, 1960.

406. Kuschinsky, G. Investigation of Sympathol, an Adrenergic Compound. Arch. exp. Path. Pharmakol. 156:290-308, 1930.

407. Mancini, M. A. The Pharmacology of the Autonomous System. Boll. Soc. ital. Biol. sper. 4:224-225, 1929.

408. Maxwell, R. A., et al. Concerning a Possible Action of Guanethidine (SU-5864) in Smooth Muscle. J. Pharmacol. exp. Ther. 129:24-30, 1960.

409. Randall, L. O. and G. Lehmann. Analgesic Action of 3-Hydroxy-N-Methyl Morphinan Hydrobromide (Dromoran). J. Pharmacol. exp. Ther. 99:163-170, 1950.

410. Bogdanski, D. F., et al. Pharmacological Studies with the Serotonin Precursor, 5-Hydroxytryptophan. J. Pharmacol. exp. Ther. 122:182-194, 1958.

411. Buchel, L. and J. Levy. Contribution to the Study of the Effects on the Central Nervous System of Monoamine Oxidese Inhibitors, Hydrazine-2-phenyl-3 propane (P. I. H.), Isopropylhydrazide of Isonicotinic Acid (Iproniazid), II. Influence on Potentiation of Experimental Sleep by Reserpine. Anesth. et Analg. 17:313-328, 1960.

412. Anderson, E. G. The Effects of Harmaline and 5-Hydroxytryptamine on Spinal Synaptic Transmission. Pharmacologist 5:238, 1963.

413. Cronhein, G. E. and J. T. Gourzis. Cardiovascular and Behavioral Effects of Serotonin and Related Substances in Dogs without and with Reserpine Premedications. J. Pharmacol. exp. Ther. 130:444-449, 1960.

414. Haas, H. On 3-Piperidino-1-Phenyl-1-Bicycloheptenylpropanol-(1) (Akineton). Second Report. Arch. int. Pharmacodyn. 128:204-238, 1960.

415. Read, G. W., et al. Comparison of Excited Phases after Sedatives and Tranquilizers. Psychopharmacologia 1:346-350, 1960.

416. Hughes, F. W. and E. Kopman. Influence of Pentobarbital, Hydroxyzine, Chlorpromazine, Reserpine, and Meprobamate on Choice-Discrimination Behavior in the Rat. Arch. int. Pharmacodyn. 126:158-170, 1960.

417. Hotovy, R. and J. Kopff-Walter. On the Pharmacological Properties of Perphenazinsulfoxide. Arzneimittel-Forsch. 10:638-650, 1960.

418. Lynes, T. E. and F. M. Berger. Some Pharmacological Properties of Hydroxyzine (1-(p-Chlorobenzhydryl-4-(2-(2-Hydroxyethoxy)-ethyl) Diethylenediamine Dihydrochloride). J. Pharmacol. exp. Ther. 119:163, 1957.

419. Hutcheon, E., et al. Cardiovascular Actions of Hydroxyzine (Atarax). J. Pharmacol. exp. Ther. 118:451-460, 1956.

420. Blackmore, W. P. Effect of Hydroxyzine on Urine Flow in the Dog. Proc. Soc. exp. Biol. (N. Y.) 103:518-520, 1960.

421. Randall, L. O. and T. H. Smith. The Adrenergic Blocking Action of Some Dibenzazepine Derivatives. J. Pharmacol. exp. Ther. 103: 10-23, 1951.

422. Cotton, M., et al. A Comparison of the Effectiveness of Adrenergic Blocking Drugs in Inhibiting the Cardiac Actions of Sympathomimetic Amines. J. Pharmacol. exp. Ther. 121:183-190, 1957.

423. Frommel, E., et al. On the Pharmacology of a New Neuroleptic: The Alpha-isomer of 2-chloro-9 (3-dimethylaminopropylidene)-Thioxanthene or Taractan; Action on Sleep Centers, on Motor Excitation Due to Nikethamide, on Pentetrazol, Electroshock and Psychomotor Excitation Due to Amphetamine. C. R. Soc. Biol. (Paris) 154:1182-1185, 1960.

424. Oberholzer, R. J. H. Experimental Data on Iminodibenzyl Derivative: Tofranil. J. Med. (Porto.) 42:602-605, 1960.

425. Dobkin, A. B. Potentiation of Thiopental Anesthesia by Derivatives and Analogs of Phenothiazine. Anesthesiology 21:292-296, 1960.

426. Gokhale, S., et al. Mechanism of the Initial Adrenergic Effects of Bretylium and Guanethidine. Brit. J. Pharmacol. 20:362-377, 1963.

427. Gyermek, L. and C. Possemato. Potentiation of 5-Hydroxytryptamine by Imipramine. Med. exp. (Basel) 3:225-229, 1960.

428. Benson, W. M., et al. Pharmacologic and Toxicologic Observations on Hydrazine Derivatives of Isonicotinic Acid (Rimifon, Marsilid). Amer. Rev. Tuberc. 65:376-391, 1952.

429. Randall, L. O. and R. E. Bagdon. Pharmacology of Iproniazid and Other Amine Oxidase Inhibitors. Ann. N. Y. Acad. Sci. 80:626-642, 1959.

430. Spector, S., et al. Biochemical and Pharmacological Effects of the Monoamine Oxidase Inhibitors, Iproniazid, 1-Phenyl-2-Hydrazinopropane (JB 516) and 1-Phenyl-3-Hydrazinobutane (JB 835). J. Pharmacol. exp. Ther. 128:15-21, 1960.

431. Bartlet, A. L. The 5-Hydroxytryptamine Content of Mouse Brain and Whole Mice after Treatment with Some Drugs Affecting the Central Nervous System. Brit. J. Pharmacol. 15:140-146, 1960.

432. Wirth, W., et al. On Testing Stimulating Substances (Hydrazine Derivatives) on "Annoyed" Animals. Arch. exp. Path. Pharmakol. 238:62-66, 1960.

433. Green, H. and R. W. Erickson. Effect of Trans-2-Phenylcyclopropylamine upon Norepinephrine Concentration and Monoamine Oxidase Activity of Rat Brain. J. Pharmacol. exp. Ther. 129:237-242, 1960.

434. Spector, S. Effect of Iproniazid on Brain Levels of Norepinephrine and Serotonin. Science 127:704, 1958.

435. Benson, W. M., et al. Comparative Pharmacology of Levorphan, Racemorphan and Dextrorphon and Related Methyl Ethers. J. Pharmacol. exp. Ther. 109:189-200, 1953.

436. Hunter, A. R. The Toxicity of Xylocaine. Brit. J. Anaesth. 23:153-161, 1951.

437. Goldberg, L. Studies on Local Anesthetics. Pharmacological Properties of Homologues and Isomers of Xylocain (Alkyl Amino-Acid Derivatives). Acta physiol. scand. 18:1-18, 1949.

438. Sorel, L. and R. Lejeune. EEG Changes in the Rabbit Following Intravenous Injection of Cocaine. Arch. int. Pharmacodyn. 102:314-334, 1955.

439. Kovalev, I. E. On the Influence of Mezocaine and Zylocaine on the Central Nervous System. Farmikol. i Toksikol. 23:385-390, 1960.

440. Bernard, C. G., et al. On the Evaluation of the Anticonvulsive Effect of Different Local Anesthetics. Arch. int. Pharmacodyn. 108:392-401, 1956.

441. Wagers, P. W. and C. M. Smith. Responses in Dental Nerves of Dogs to Tooth Stimulation and the Effects of Systemically Administered Procaine, Lidocaine and Morphine. J. Pharmacol. exp. Ther. 130:89-105, 1960.

442. Bernhard, C. G., et al. The Difference in Action on Normal and Convulsive Cortical Activity between a Local Anesthetic (Lidocaine) and Barbiturate. Arch. int. Pharmacodyn. 108:408-419, 1956.

443. Gogerty, J. and J. Dille. Pharmacology of d-Lysergic-Acid Morpholide (LSM). J. Pharmacol. exp. Ther. 120:340-348, 1957.

444. Delphant, J. and M. Lanza. Comparative Action of Mescaline, LSD 25, and Yajeine on the Central Temperature of the Rat. J. Physiol. (Paris) 52:70-71, 1960.

445. Weltman, A. S., et al. Endocrine Effects of Lysergic Acid Diethylamide on Male Rats. Fed. Proc. 22:165, 1963.

446. Yui, T. and Y. Takeo. Neuropharmacological Studies on a New Series of Ergot Alkaloids. Jap. J. Pharmacol. 7:157-161, 1958.

447. Key, B. J. and P. B. Bradley. The Effects of Drugs on Conditioning and Habituation to Arousal Stimuli in Animals. Psychopharmacologia 1:450-462, 1960.

448. Passonant, P., et al. The Action of LSD-25 on the Behavior and on the Cortical and Rhinencephalic Rhythms of the Chronic Cat. Electroenceph. clin. Neurophysiol. 8:702, 1956.

449. Apter, J. T. LSD-25 Versus Pentobarbital Sodium. Fed. Proc. 17:5, 1958.

450. Elder, J. T. Phenoxybenzamine (PBA) Antagonism of Lysergic Acid Diethylamide (LSD)-Induced Hyperglycemia. Pharmacologist 5:261, 1963.

451. Dobkin, A. B. and J. H. Havland. Drugs Which Stimulate Affective Behavior. I. Action of Lysergic Acid Diethylamide (LSD-25) Against

Thiopentone Anesthesia in Dogs. Anaesthesia 15:48-54, 1960.

452. Murray, E. J. and S. Chorover. Effects of Lysergic Acid Diethylamine upon Certain Aspects of Memory (Delayed Alternation) in Monkeys. Fed. Proc. 17:381, 1958.

453. Weidmann, H. and A. Cerletti. Investigation of the Pressor Activity of 5-Hydroxytryptamine (Serotonin). Arch. int. Pharmacodyn. 111:98-107, 1957.

454. Meltzer, S. J. and J. Auer. Physiological and Pharmacological Studies of Magnesium Salts. I. General Anesthesia by Subcutaneous Injections. Amer. J. Physiol. 14:366-388, 1905.

455. Gylus, J. A., et al. Pharmacological and Toxicological Properties of 2-Methyl-3-Piperidinopyrazine, a New Antidepressant. Ann. N. Y. Acad. Sci. 107:899-912, 1963.

456. Heise, G. A. and E. Boff. Behavioral Determination of Time and Dose Parameters of Monoamine Oxidase Inhibitors. J. Pharmacol. exp. Ther. 129:155-162, 1960.

457. Berger, F. M., et al. The Pharmacological Properties of 2-Methyl-2-Sec-Butyl-1,3-Propanediol Dicarbamate (Mebutamate, W-583), a New Centrally Acting Blood Pressure Lowering Agent. J. Pharmacol. exp. Ther. 134:356-365, 1961.

458. Rowe, G. G., et al. The Effect of Mecamylamine on Coronary Flow, Cardiac Work and Cardiac Efficiency in Normotensive Dogs. J. Lab. clin. Med. 52:883-887, 1958.

459. Lum, B. K. B. and P. L. Rushleigh. Potentiation of Vasoactive Drugs by Ganglionic Blocking Agents. J. Pharmacol. exp. Ther. 132:13-18, 1961.

460. Lakeside Laboratories. Personal Communication.

461. Roszkowski, A. P. A Pharmacological Comparison of Therapeutically Useful Centrally Acting Skeletal Muscle Relaxants. J. Pharmacol. exp. Ther. 129:75-81, 1960.

462. Burke, J. C., et al. The Muscle Relaxant Properties of 2,2-Dichloro-1-(p-Chlorophenyl)-1,3-Propanediol-O^3-Carbamate. Arch. int. Pharmacodyn. 134:216-223, 1961.

463. Della Bella, D. and F. Rognoni. Pharmacologic Properties of a New Synthetic Derivative with Central Depressant Activity: 2-2-bis-Chloromethyl-1, 3-Propanediol (Dispranol). Boll. chim. farm. 99:67-78, 1960.

464. Seifter, J., et al. Pharmacology of N-Methyl-ω-Phenyl-Tert-Butylamine. 116th Meeting Am. Chem. Soc. 17L, 1949.

465. Day, M. D. Effect of Sympathomimetic Amines on the Blocking Action of Guanethidine, Bretylium and Xylocholine. Brit. J. Pharmacol. 18:421-439, 1962.

466. Covino, B. G. Antifibrillary Effect of Mephentermine Sulfate (Wyamine) in General Hypothermia. J. Pharmacol. exp. Ther. 122:418-422, 1958.

467. Brofman, B. L., et al. Treatment of Hypotension Accompanying Myocardial Infarction: Use of a Pressor Substance. J. Lab. clin. Med. 36:802, 1950.

468. Fawaz, G. The Effect of Mephentermine on Isolated Dog Hearts, Normal and Pretreated with Reserpine. Brit. J. Pharmacol. 16:309-314, 1961.

469. Aston, R. and H. Cullumbine. The Effects of Combinations of Ataraxics with Hypnotics, LSD and Iproniozid in the Mouse. Arch. int. Pharmacodyn. 126:219-227, 1960.

470. Geller, I. and J. Seifter. The Effects of Meprobamate, Barbiturates, d-Amphetamine and Promazine on Experimentally Induced Conflict in the Rat. Psychopharmacologia (Berl.) 1:482-492, 1960.

471. Takeda, Y. Pharmacological and Toxicological Studies on Tranquilizers. Yakugaku Kenkyu 32:585-616, 1960.

472. Ledebur, I. v., et al. Nalorphine Antagonism of the Narcotic Action of Chlorpromazine, Meprobamate, and Methaminodiazepoxide (Librium). Med. Exptl. 7:177-179, 1962.

473. Hendley, C. D., et al. Effects of Meprobamate (Miltown), Chlorpromazine, and Reserpine on Behavior in the Monkey. Fed. Proc. 15:436, 1956.

474. Barnes, T. C. Effects of Tranquilizers and Antiepileptic Drugs on EEG-Flicker Response and on Convulsive Behavior. Fed. Proc. 17:347, 1958.

475. Orth, O. S., et al. Subacute Toxicity of

"Thiomerin" Compared to Other Mercurial Diuretics. Fed. Proc. 9:305-306, 1950.

476. Ernst, A. M. Experiments with an O-Methylated Product of Dopamine on Cats. Acta physiol. pharmacol. neerl. 11:48-53, 1962.

477. Parker, J. M. and N. Hildebrand. Mescaline Blocking Effects of Dibenamine. Fed. Proc. 21:419, 1962.

478. Hosko, M. J., Jr. and R. Tislow. Acute Tolerance to Mescaline in the Dog. Fed. Proc. 15:440, 1956.

479. Bridger, W. H. and W. H. Gantt. The Effect of Mescaline on Differentiated Conditional Reflexes. Amer. J. Psychiat. 113:352-360, 1956.

480. Chen, K. K. Pharmacology of Methadone and Related Compounds. Ann. N. Y. Acad. Sci. 51:83-97, 1948.

481. Finnegan, J. K., et al. Observations on the Comparative Pharmacologic Actions of 6-Dimethylamino-4, 4-Diphenyl-3-Heptanone (Amidone) and Morphine. J. Pharmacol. exp. Ther. 92:269-276, 1948.

482. Eddy, N. B. and D. Leimbach. Synthetic Analgesics. II. Dithienylbutenyl and Dithienylbutylamines. J. Pharmacol. exp. Ther. 107:385-393, 1953.

483. Holten, C. H. and E. Sonne. Action of a Series of Benactyzine-Derivatives and Other Compounds on Stress-Induced Behavior in the Rat. Acta pharmacol. (Kbh.) 11:148-155, 1955.

484. Somers, G. F. Pharmacological Properties of Thalidomide (α-Phtyalimido Glutarmide), a New Sedative Hypnotic Drug. Brit. J. Pharmacol. 15:111-116, 1960.

485. Hauschild, F. The Pharmacology of Phenylalkylamine. Arch. exp. Path. Pharmakol. 195:647-680, 1940.

486. Owen, J. E., Jr. The Influence of dl, d- and 1-Amphetamine and d-Methamphetamine on a Fixed-Ratio Schedule. J. exp. Anal. Behav. 3:293-310, 1960.

487. John, E. R., et al. Differential Effects on Various Conditioned Responses in Cats Caused by Intraventricular and Intramuscular Injections of Reserpine and Other Substances. J. Pharmacol. exp. Ther. 123:193-205, 1958.

488. Hjort, A. M., et al. The Pharmacology of Compounds Related to β-2, 5-Dimethoxy, Phenethyl Amine. J. Pharmacol. exp. Ther. 92:283-290, 1948.

489. De Beer, E. J., et al. The Restoration of Arterial Pressure from Various Hypotensive States by Methoxamine. Arch. int. Pharmacodyn. 104:487-498, 1956.

490. Stormorken, H., et al. Mechanism of Bradycardia by Methoxamine. Arch. int. Pharmacodyn. 120:386-401, 1959.

491. Visscher, F. E., et al. Pharmacology of Pamine Bromide. J. Pharmacol. exp. Ther. 110:188-204, 1954.

492. Smith, S. E. The Pharmacological Actions of 3-4-Dihydroxyphenyl-α-Methylamine (α-Methyldopa), an Inhibitor of 5-Hydroxytryptophan Decarboxylase. Brit. J. Pharmacol. 15:319-327, 1960.

493. Dangler, H. and G. Reichel. Inhibition of Dopa Decarboxylase by 2-Methyl-3-(3, 4-Dihydroxyphenyl) Alanine (α-methyl Dopa) in vivo. Arch. exp. Path. Pharmakol. 234:275-281, 1958.

494. Westermann, E., et al. Inhibition of Serotonin Formation by α-Methyl-3, 4-Dihydroxyphenyl-L-Alanine. Arch. exp. Path. Pharmakol. 234:194-205, 1958.

495. Sergio, C. and V. G. Longo. Action of Several Drugs on EEG and Behavior of Decorticate Rabbits. Arch. int. Pharmacodyn. 125:65-82, 1960.

496. Maxwell, R. A., et al. Differential Potentiation of Norepinephrine and Epinephrine by Cardiovascular and CNS-Active Agents. J. Pharmacol. exp. Ther. 128:140-144, 1960.

497. Maxwell, R. A., et al. Studies Concerning the Cardiovascular Actions of the Central Nervous Stimulant, Methylphenidate. J. Pharmacol. exp. Ther. 123:22-27, 1958.

498. Maxwell, R. A., et al. A Comparison of Some of the Cardiovascular Actions of Methylphenidate and Cocaine. J. Pharmacol. exp. Ther. 126:250-257, 1959.

499. Eddy, N. B. Pharmacology of Metopon and Other New Analgesic Opium Derivatives. Ann. N. Y. Acad. Sci. 51:51-58, 1948.

500. Chesler, A., et al. A Study of the Comparative Toxic Effects of Morphine on the Fetal,

Newborn and Adult Rat. J. Pharmacol. exp. Ther. 75:363-366, 1942.

501. Haag, H. B., et al. Pharmacologic Observations on 1,1-Diphenyl-1-(dimethylaminoisopropyl)-butanone-2. Fed. Proc. 6:334, 1947.

502. Hatcher, R. A. and C. Eggleston. Studies on the Absorption of Drugs. J. Amer. med. Ass. 63:(1):469-473, 1914.

503. Himmelsbach, C. K., et al. A Method for Testing Addiction, Tolerance and Abstinence in the Rat. J. Pharmacol. exp. Ther. 53:179-188, 1935.

504. Blozovski, M. and J. Jacob. The Effect of Morphine on the Behavior of Mice Trained to Run through an Elevated Maze. Arch. int. Pharmacodyn. 124:422-435, 1960.

505. Olds, H., and R. P. Travis. Effects of Chlorpromazine, Meprobamate, Pentobarbital and Morphine on Self-Stimulation. J. Pharmacol. exp. Ther. 128:397-404, 1960.

506. Tedeschi, D. H., et al. Analgesic and Other Neuropharmacologic Effects of Phenazocine (NIH 7519, Prinadol) Compared with Morphine. J. Pharmacol. exp. Ther. 130:431-435, 1960.

507. Zirm, K. L. and A. Pongratz. The Analgetic Action of the Pyridin-3-Carbonic Acid Bis Ester of Morphine. Arzneimittel-Forsch. 10: 137-139, 1960.

508. Wright, C. I. and F. A. Barbour. The Respiratory Effects of Morphine, Codeine and Related Substances. J. Pharmacol. exp. Ther. 53:34-45, 1935.

509. Longo, V. G. Electroencephalographic Atlas for Pharmacological Research. Elsevier Publ. Co., New York and Amsterdam, 1962.

510. Takagi, H., et al. The Effect of Analgesics on the Spinal Reflex Activity of the Cat. Jap. J. Pharmacol. 4:176-187, 1955.

511. Führer, H. Pharmacological Actions of Muscarine Derivatives. Arch. exp. Path. Pharm. 61:283-296, 1909.

512. Mattila, M. and P. Lavikainen. The Mouse Tail Reaction Induced by Morphine and the Sedative Action after Reserpine and Nalorphine. Ann. Med. exp. Fenn. 38:115-120, 1960.

513. Hart, E. R. and E. L. McCawley. The Pharmacology of N-Allylnormorphine as Compared

with Morphine. J. Pharmacol. exp. Ther. 182:339-348, 1944.

514. Kirvoy, W. A. and R. A. Huggins. The Action of Morphine, Methadone, Meperidine and Nalorphine on Dorsal Root Potentials of Cat Spinal Cord. J. Pharmacol. exp. Ther. 134:210-213, 1961.

515. Unna, K. Antagonistic Effect of N-Allyl-Normorphine upon Morphine. J. Pharmacol. exp. Ther. 79:27-31, 1943.

516. Goldstein, L. and J. Aldunate. Quantitative Electroencephalographic Studies of the Effects of Morphine and Nalorphine on Rabbit Brain. J. Pharmacol. exp. Ther. 130:204-211, 1960.

517. Brown, B. B., et al. A Comparative Study of Tetramethoquin, a New Parasympathetic Stimulant, Neostigmine and Physostigmine. Arch. int. Pharmacodyn. 81:276-289, 1950.

518. Haley, T. J. and B. M. Rhodes. A Note on the Acute Toxicity of Neostigmine Methyl Bromide in the Rat. J. Am. pharm. Ass. 39: 701, 1950.

519. Aeschlimann, J. A. and M. Reinert. The Pharmacological Action of Some Analogues of Physostigmine. J. Pharmacol. exp. Ther. 43:413-444, 1931.

520. Heathcote, R. St. A. The Pharmacological Action of Eseridine. J. Pharmacol. exp. Ther. 46:375-385, 1932.

521. Polonovski, M. and M. Polonovski. Alkaloidal Derivatives with Attenuated Toxicity. C. R. Acad. Sci. (Paris) 181:887-888, 1925.

522. Carlsson, A. and N. Hillarp. Formation of Phenolic Acids in Brain After Administration of 3,4-Dihydroxyphenylalanine. Acta physiol. scand. 55:95-100, 1962.

523. P'an, S. Y., et al. Anticonvulsant Effect of Nialamide and Diphenylhydantoin. Proc. Soc. 108:680-683, 1961.

524. Larson, P. S., et al. Studies on the Fate of Nicotine in the Body. VI. Observations on the Relative Rate of Elimination of Nicotine by the Dog, Cat, Rabbit and Mouse. J. Pharmacol. exp. Ther. 95:506-508, 1949.

525. Heubner, W. and J. Papierkowski. On the Toxicity of Nicotine in Mice. Arch. exp. Path. Pharmakol. 188:605-610, 1938.

526. Behrend, A. and C. H. Thienes. The Development of Tolerance to Nicotine by Rats. J. Pharmacol. exp. Ther. 48:317-325, 1933.

527. Chen, K. K., et al. Toxicity of Nicotinic Acid. Proc. Soc. exp. Biol. (N. Y.) 38:241-245, 1938.

528. Hatcher, R. A. Nicotine Tolerance in Rabbits and the Difference in the Total Dose in Adult and Young Guinea Pigs. Amer. J. Physiol. 11:17-27, 1904.

529. Bonta, I. L., et al. A Newly Developed Motility Apparatus and its Applicability in Two Pharmacological Designs. Arch. int. Pharmacodyn. 129:381-394, 1960.

530. Hardt, A. and R. Hotovy. Methods of Testing for Compounds with Curare-Like Action. Arch. exp. Path. Pharmakol. 209:264-278, 1950.

531. Smith, C. S., et al. Study of the Effect of Nicotinism in the Albino Rat. J. Pharmacol. exp. Ther. 55:274-287, 1935.

532. Kuschinsky, G. and R. Hotovy. On the Central Stimulative Action of Nicotine. Klin. Wschr. 22:649-650, 1943.

533. Knapp, D. E. and E. F. Comino. Evidence for a Nicotinic Receptor in the Central Nervous System Related to EEG Arousal. Fed. Proc. 20:307, 1961.

534. Novikova, A. A. Influence of Nicotine upon Reflex Activity. Bull. eksp. Biol. Med. S.S.S.R. 9:38-42, 1940.

535. Schaepdryver, A. F. de. Hypertensive Responses in Reserpinized Dogs. Arch. int. Pharmacodyn. 124:45-52, 1960.

536. Behrens, B. and E. Reichelt. A Comparison of Cardiazol and Coramin in an Animal Experiment. Klin. Wschr. 12:1860-1862, 1933.

537. Hildebrandt, F. Pentamethylentetrazol (Cardiazol). Heffter's Hdb. E. 5:151-183, 1937.

538. Albus, G. Animal Experiments with Commercial Stimulants with Particular Consideration of Cardiazole and Coramine. Arch. int. Path. Pharmakol. 182:471-476, 1936.

539. Eichholtz, F. and T. Kirsch. The Effect of Depressor Substances on Cocaine Convulsions. Arch. exp. Path. Pharmakol. 184:674-679, 1937.

540. Heubner, W. and A. v. Nyary. Cumulation of the Digitalis Glucosides. Arch. exp. Path. Pharmakol. 177:60-73, 1934.

541. White, A. C. The Pharmacological and Toxic Action of Digoxin. J. Pharmacol. exp. Ther. 52:1-22, 1934.

542. Boyajy, L. D. and C. B. Nash. Influence of Reserpine on Fibrillatory and Positive Inotropic Responses to Ouabain. Fed. Proc. 22:185, 1963.

543. Henderson, F. G., et al. Pharmacologic Studies of 6,7-Dimethoxy, 1-(4'-ethoxy-3'-methoxybenzyl)3-Methyl-Isoquinoline. J. Amer. pharm. Ass. 40:207, 1951.

544. Macht, D. I. A Pharmacologic and Clinical Study of Papaverin. Arch. intern. Med. 17:786-805, 1916.

545. Leopold-Lowenthal, H. On the Pharmacological Properties of 1-Methyl-butyl-2-Phenyl-2-Hydroxypropionate (Spasmol). Wien med. Wschr. 101:61, 1951.

546. Drommond, F. G., et al. Toxicity of Some Opium Alkaloids. Acta pharmacol. (Kbh.) 6:235-249, 1950.

547. Tunger, H. The Duration of Narcosis and the Narcotic Range of Nonspecific Narcotics in Different Methods of Administration. Arch. exp. Path. Pharmakol. 160:74-91, 1931.

548. Figot, P. P., et al. The Estimation and Significance of Paraldehyde Levels in Blood and Brain. Acta pharmacol. (Kbh.) 8:290-304, 1952.

549. Kay, F. A., et al. Studies on Paraldehyde. I. The Median Lethal Dose, LD_{50}, of Paraldehyde for Guinea Pigs. Anesthesiology 5:182-185, 1944.

550. Jenney, E. H. and C. C. Pfeiffer. The Convulsant Effect of Hydrazides and the Antidotal Effect of Anticonvulsants and Metabolites. J. Pharmacol. exp. Ther. 122:110-123, 1958.

551. Everett, G. M. Pharmacologic Studies of Some Nonhydrazine MAO Inhibitors. Ann. N. Y. Acad. Sci. 107:1068-1077, 1963.

552. Spector, S. Monoamine Oxidase in Control of Brain Serotonin and Norepinephrine Content. Ann. N. Y. Acad. Sci. 107:856-861, 1963.

553. Schoepke, H. G. and R. G. Wiegand. Relation between Norepinephrine Accumulation or Depletion and Blood Pressure Responses in the Cat and Rat Following Pargyline Administration. Ann. N. Y. Acad. Sci. 107:924-934, 1963.

554. Taylor, J. D., et al. A New Non-Hydrazide Monoamine Oxidase Inhibitor (A 19120) (N-Methyl-N-Benzyl-2-Propynylamine Hydrochloride). Fed. Proc. 19:278, 1960.

555. Calesnick, B. et al. Combined Action of Cardiotoxic Drugs: A Study on the Acute Toxicity of Combined Quinidine, Meperidine, Pentobarbital, Procaine, and Procaine Amide. J. Pharmacol. exp. Ther. 102:138-143, 1951.

556. Carmichael, E. B. and L. C. Posey. Toxicity of Nembutal for Guinea Pigs. Proc. Soc. exp. Biol. (N.Y.) 33:527-528, 1936.

557. Westhues, M. and R. Fritsch. The Narcosis of Animals. Paul Parcy, Berlin, 1961.

558. Krop, S. and H. Gold. Comparative Study of Several Barbiturates with Observations on Irreversible Neurological Disturbances. J. Pharmacol. exp. Ther. 88:260-267, 1946.

559. White, R. P. and L. D. Boyajy. Comparison of Physostigmine and Amphetamine in Antagonizing the Electroencephalogram (EEG) Effects of Central Nervous System Depressants. Proc. Soc. exp. Biol. (N.Y.) 102:479-483, 1959.

560. Schallek, W., et al. Central Depressant Effects of Methyprylon. J. Pharmacol. exp. Ther. 118:139-147, 1956.

561. Kneip, P. Climbing Impulse and Climbing Test. Arch. int. Pharmacodyn. 126:238-245, 1960.

562. Tsobkallo, G. I. and M. K. Kalinina. Effect of Barbamyl, Nembutal and Thiopental on the Higher Nervous Activity of Rabbits. Pavlov J. High. Nerv. Act. 10:644-652, 1960.

563. Bradley, P. B. and B. J. Key. The Effect of Drugs on Arousal Responses Produced by Electrical Stimulation of the Reticular Formation. Electroenceph. clin. Neurophysiol. 10:97-110, 1958.

564. Pfeiffer, C. C., et al. Comparative Study of the Effect of Meprobamate on the Conditioned Response, on Strychnine and Pentenetetrazol Thresholds, on the Normal Electroencephalogram, and on Polysynaptic Reflexes. Ann. N. Y. Acad. Sci. 67:734-743, 1957.

565. Martin, W. R. and C. G. Eades. A Comparative Study of the Effect of Drugs on Activation and Vasomotor Responses Evoked by Midbrain Stimulation: Atropine, Pentobarbital, Chlorpromazine and Chlorpromazine Sulfoxide. Psychopharmacologia 1:303-335, 1960.

566. Abdulian, D. H., et al. Effects of Central Nervous System Depressants on Inhibition And Facilitation of the Patellar Reflex. Arch. int. Pharmacodyn. 128:169-186, 1960.

567. Mitchell, J. C. and F. A. King. The Effects of Chlorpromazine on Water Maze Learning Retention, and Stereotyped Behavior in the Rat. Psychopharmacologia 1:463-468, 1960.

568. Domer, F. R. and W. Feldberg. The Effect of Administration of Drugs into the Cerebral Ventricles. Brit. J. Pharmacol. 15:578-587, 1960.

569. McOmie, W. A. Local and Systemic Effects of 2-Methyl 2,4-Pentanedial (Hexylene Glycol). Fed. Proc. 6:357, 1947.

570. Hildebrandt, F. Pyridin-β-Carboxylic Acid Diethylamide (Coramin). Heffter's Hdb. E.5: 128-150.

571. Gross, E. G. and R. M. Featherstone. Studies with Tetrazole Derivatives. I. Some Pharmacologic Properties of Aliphatic Substitutes Pentamethylene Tetrazole Derivatives. J. Pharmacol. exp. Ther. 87:291-305, 1946.

572. Werner, H. W. and A. L. Tatum. A Comparative Study of the Stimulant Analeptics Picrotoxin, Metrazol and Coramine. J. Pharmacol. exp. Ther. 66:260-278, 1939.

573. Ziph, K., et al. The Antagonistic Action of Cardiazole, Coramine, Hexetone, Strychnine and Icoral to Narcotics. Arch. exp. Path. Pharmakol. 185:113-124, 1937.

574. Hildebrandt, F. and J. Voss. Absorption of Cardiazol Following Oral Administration. München med. Wchnschr. 73:862, 1926.

575. Chusid, J. and L. Kopeloff. Chlordiazepoxide as an Anticonvulsant in Monkeys. Proc. Soc. exp. Biol. (N.Y.) 109:546-548, 1962.

576. Wallace, G. D., et al. Restraint of Chimpanzees with Perphenazine. J. Am. vet. med. Ass. 136:222-224, 1960.

577. High, J. P., et al. Pharmacology of Fluphenazine (Prolixin). Toxicol. appl. Pharmacol. 2: 540-552, 1960.

578. Taeschler, M., et al. On the Significance of Various Pharmacodynamic Properties of Phenothiazine Derivatives for their Clinical Effectiveness. Psychiat. et Neurol. (Basel) 139:85-104, 1960.

579. Scott, C. C., et al. Comparison of the Pharmacologic Properties of Some New Analgesic Substances. Curr. Res. Anesth. 26:12-17, 1947.

580. Gruber, C. M. and E. R. Hart. The Pharmacology and Toxicology of the Ethyl Ester of 1-Methyl-4-Phenyl-Piperidine-4-Carboxylic Acid (Demerol). J. Pharmacol. exp. Ther. 73:319-334, 1941.

581. Foster, R. H. K. and A. L. Carman. Studies in Analgesia: Piperidine Derivatives with Morphine-Like Activity. J. Pharmacol. exp. Ther. 91:195-209, 1947.

582. Emele, J. F., et al. The Analgesic Activity of Phenelzine and Other Compounds. J. Pharmacol. exp. Ther. 134:206-209, 1961.

583. Ben, M., et al. Cardiovascular Activity of β-Phenylethylhydrazine (Phenelzine). Angiology 11:62-66, 1960.

584. Eltherington, L. G. and A. Horita. Some Pharmacological Actions of Beta-Phenylisopropylhydrazine (PIH). J. Pharmacol. exp. Ther. 128:7-14, 1960.

585. Buchel, L. and J. Levy. Contribution to the Study of the Effects of Hydrazine-2-Phenyl-3-Propane (PIH) on the Central Nervous System, Compared with Those of 1-Isonicotinyl-2-Isopropylhydrazine (Iproniazid). I. Influence on Experimental Hypnosis. Anesth. et Analg. 17:289-312, 1960.

586. Buckley, J. P., et al. The Pharmacology of Beta-Phenylisopropylhydrazine. Fed. Proc. 19:278, 1960.

587. Schaffarsick, R. W. and B. J. Brown. The Anticonvulsant Activity and Toxicity of Methylparafynol (Dormison) and Some Other Alcohols. Science 116:663-665, 1952.

588. Fitch, R. H. and A. L. Tatum. The Duration of Action of the Barbituric Acid Hypnotics as a Basis of Classification. J. Pharmacol. exp. Ther. 44:325-335, 1932.

589. Anderson, E. G. and D. D. Bonnycastle. A Study of the Central Depressant Action of Pentobarbital, Phenobarbital and Diethyl Ether in Relationship to Increases in Brain 5-Hydroxytryptamine. J. Pharmacol. exp. Ther. 130:138-143, 1960.

590. Wilson, H. and J. P. Long. The Effect of Hemicholinium (HC-3) at Various Peripheral Cholinergic Transmitting Sites. Arch. int. Pharmacodyn. 120:343-352, 1959.

591. Bodo, R. C. de and K. F. Prescott. The Antidiuretic Action of Barbiturates (Phenobarbital, Amytal, Pentobarbital) and the Mechanism Involved in this Action. J. Pharmacol. exp. Ther. 85:222-233, 1945.

592. Truitt, E. B., Jr., et al. Measurement of Brain Excitability by Use of Hexafluorodiethyl Ether (Indoklon). J. Pharmacol. exp. Ther. 129:445-453, 1960.

593. De Salva, S. Continuous Intravenous Infusion of Strychnine in Rats: III. Endocrine Influences. Arch. int. Pharmacodyn. 125:355-361, 1960.

594. Weaver, L. C., et al. Central Nervous System Effects of a Local Anesthetic, Dyclonine. Toxicol. appl. Pharmacol. 2:616-627, 1960.

595. Delgado, J. M. R., et al. Effect of Amphenidone on the Brain of the Conscious Monkey. Arch. int. Pharmacodyn. 125:161-171, 1960.

596. Vogel, G. and L. Ther. The Behavior of the Cotton Rat as Determinant of Neuroleptic Ratio of Central-Depressing Compounds. Arzneimittel-Forsch. 10:806-808, 1960.

597. Domino, E. F., et al. Differential Effects of Some CNS Depressants on a Quantitative Shock Avoidance Response in the Dog. J. Pharmacol. exp. Ther. 122:20A, 1958.

598. Scheer, E. The Depressant Effect of Sodium Ethylcrotyl Barbiturate on the Central Nervous System and Influences on Blood Pressure and Blood Sugar. Acta Biol. et Med. Ger. 5:545-560, 1960.

599. Sobek, V. Effects of Barbiturates on Reflex Peristaltic Inhibition. Farmakol. i Toksikol. 23:17-20, 1960.

600. Schapiro, S. Effect of a Catechol Amine Blocking Agent (Dibenzyline) on Organ Content and Urine Excretion of Noradrenaline and Adrenaline. Acta physiol. scand. 42:371-375, 1958.

601. Quinn, G. P., et al. Biochemical and Pharmacological Studies of RO1-9569 (Tetrabena-

zine), a Non-Indole Tranquilizing Agent with Reserpine-Like Effects. J. Pharmacol. exp. Ther. 127:103-109, 1959.

602. Innes, I. R. Identification of the Smooth Muscle Excitatory Receptors for Ergot Alkaloids. Brit. J. Pharmacol. 19:120-128, 1962.

603. Meier, R., et al. A New Imidazoline Derivative with Marked Adrenolytic Properties. Proc. Soc. exp. Biol. (N. Y.) 71:70-72, 1949.

604. Furchgott, R. F. In: Ciba Foundation Symposium, eds. Vane, J. R., et al. Little Brown, Boston, 1960, p. 246.

605. Hazleton, L. W., et al. Toxicity of Phenylbutazone (Butazolidin). Fed. Proc. 12:330, 1953.

606. Kuschinsky, G. and K. Oberdisse. Circulatory Effects of Meta-Sympatole. Arch. exp. Path. Pharm. 162:46-55, 1931.

607. Warren, M. R. and H. W. Werner. The Central Stimulant Action of Some Vasopressor Amines. J. Pharmacol. exp. Ther. 85:119-121, 1945.

608. Chessin, M., et al. Biochemical and Pharmacological Studies of β-Phenylhydrazine and Selected Related Compounds. Ann. N. Y. Acad. Sci. 80:597-608, 1959.

609. Way, E. L. Barbiturate Antagonism of Isonipecaine Convulsions and Isonipecaine Potentiation of Barbiturate Depression. J. Pharmacol. exp. Ther. 87:265-272, 1946.

610. Gruhzit, O. M. Sodium Diphenyl Hydantoinate: Pharmacologic and Histopathologic Studies. Arch. Path. 28:761-762, 1939.

611. Knoefel, P. K. and G. Lehmann. The Anticonvulsive Action of Diphenyl Hydantoin and Some Related Compounds. J. Pharmacol. exp. Ther. 72:194-201, 1942.

612. Everett, G. M. and R. K. Richards. Comparative Anti-Convulsive Action of 3, 5, 5-Trimethyloxazolidine-2, 4-Dione (Tridione), Dilantin and Phenobarbital. J. Pharmacol. exp. Ther. 81:402-407, 1944.

613. Esplin, D. W. and J. W. Freston. Physiological and Pharmacological Analysis of Spinal Cord Convulsions. J. Pharmacol. exp. Ther. 130:68-80, 1960.

614. Heubner, W. Pharmacological and Chemical Investigation of Physostigmine. Arch. exp. Path. Pharmakol. 53:313-330, 1905.

615. Zetler, G., et al. Research Toward a Pharmacological Differentiation of Cataleptic Effects. Arch. exp. Path. Pharmakol. 238:468-501, 1960.

616. Hjort, A. M. and E. J. deBeer. The Effect of the Diet upon the Anesthetic Qualities of Some Hypnotics. J. Pharmacol. exp. Ther. 65:79-88, 1939.

617. Swanson, E. E. and K. K. Chen. The Pharmacological Action of Coriamyrtin. J. Pharmacol. exp. Ther. 57:410-418, 1936.

618. Apter, J. T. Analeptic Action of Lysergic Acid Diethylamide (LSD-25) Against Pentobarbital. Arch. Neurol. Psychiat. (Chic.) 79:711-715, 1958.

619. Holck, H. G. O. and P. R. Cannon. On the Cause of the Delayed Death in the Rat by Isopropyl Betabromallyl Barbituric Acid (Nostal) and Some Related Barbiturates. J. Pharmacol. exp. Ther. 57:289-309, 1936.

620. Zablocka, B. and D. W. Esplin. Central Excitatory and Depressant Effects of Pilocarpine in Rats and Mice. J. Pharmacol. exp. Ther. 140:162-169, 1963.

621. Singh, S. D. and H. J. Eysenck. Conditioned Emotional Response in the Rat. III. Drug Antagonism. J. Gen. Psychol. 63:275-285, 1960.

622. Stone, G. C. Effects of Some Centrally Acting Drugs upon Learning of Escape and Avoidance Habits. J. comp. physiol. Psychol. 53:33-37, 1960.

623. Larson, R. E. and G. L. Plaa. Effect of Spinal Cord Transection on CCl_4 Hepatotoxicity. Fed. Proc. 22:189, 1963.

624. Gettler, A. O. and J. Baine. The Toxicology of Cyanide. Amer. J. med. Sci. 195:182-188, 1938.

625. Lindgren, P. and A. Sundwall. Parasympatholytic Effects of TMB-4 (1, 1-Trimethylenebis (4-Formylpyridinium Bromide)-Dioxime) and Some Related Oximes in the Cat. Acta pharmacol. (Kbh.) 17:69-83, 1960.

626. Santi, R., et al. Pharmacological Action of N, N-Diisopropylammonium Dichloroacetate (DIEDI). Minerva Med. 51, Suppl. 71:2909-2919, 1960.

627. McKinney, S. E., et al. Benemid, p-(D1-n-Propylsulamyl)-Benzoic Acid: Toxicologic Properties. J. Pharmacol. exp. Ther. 102: 208-214, 1951.

628. Seiffer, J. et al. The Toxicity of N, N'-Dibenzylethylenediamine (DBED) and DBED Dipenecillin. Antibiot. et Chemother. (Basel) 1: 504-508, 1951.

629. Naranjo, P. and E. B. de Naranjo. Local Anesthetic Activity of Some Antihistamines and its Relationship with the Antihistaminic and Anticholinergic Activities. Arch. int. Pharmacodyn. 113:313-335, 1958.

630. Richards, R. K. and K. E. Kueter. Competitive Inhibition of Procaine Convulsions in Guinea Pigs. J. Pharmacol. exp. Ther. 87:42-52, 1946.

631. Schneider, J. A. and F. F. Yonkman. Species Differences in the Respiratory and Cardiovascular Response to Serotonin (5-Hydroxytryptamine). J. Pharmacol. exp. Ther. 111:84-98, 1954.

632. Ilyuchenok, R. Y. Comparative Study of the Influence of Chlorpromazine and Propazine on the Bioelectric Activity of the Cerebrum. Zh. Nevopat. Psikhiat. 60:202-209, 1960.

633. Ekstrom, N. and F. Sandberg. A Method for Quantitative Determination of the Inhibitory Action on C. A. R. of Mice. Arzneimittel-Forsch. 12:1208-1209, 1962.

634. Schneider, J. A. Further Characterization of Central Effects of Reserpine (Serpasil). Am. J. Physiol. 181:64-68, 1955.

635. Innes, I. R. Sensitization of the Heart and Nictitating Membrane of the Cat to Sympathomimetic Amines by Antihistamine Drugs. Brit. J. Pharmacol. 13:6-10, 1958.

636. Black, J. W. and J. S. Stephenson. Pharmacology of a New Adrenergic Beta-Receptor Blocking Compound (Nethalide). Lancet 2: 311-314, 18 Aug., 1962.

637. Goldberg, M. E. and G. V. Rossi. The Effect of Anticholinergic Compounds on Several Components of Gastric Secretion in Pylorus-Ligated Rats. J. Amer. pharm. Ass. 49:543-547, 1960.

638. Abbott, C. E. B., et al. Effect of Propantheline Bromide (Pro-Banthine) on Fluid and Electrolyte Loss in Dogs with Pyloric Obstruc-tion. Canad. med. Ass. J. 76:176-180, 1957.

639. Krayer, O., et al. Studies on Veratrum Alkaloids. VI. Protoveratrine: Its Comparative Toxicity and its Circulatory Action. J. Pharmacol. exp. Ther. 82:167-186, 1944.

640. Swiss, E. D. and R. O. Bauer. Acute Toxicity of Veratrum Derivatives. Proc. Soc. exp. Biol. (N. Y.) 76:847-849, 1951.

641. Haas, H. T. A. Pharmacology of Germerine and its Degradation Products. I. Arch. exp. Path. Pharmakol. 189:397-410, 1938.

642. Martini, L. and L. Calliauw. On the Pharmacology of Protoveratrine in Dogs. Arch. int. Pharmacodyn. 101:49-67, 1955.

643. Mosey, L. and A. Kaplan. Respiratory Effects of Potent Hypotensive Derivatives of Veratrum. J. Pharmacol. exp. Ther. 104: 67-75, 1952.

644. Woolley, D. W. and N. K. Campbell. Serotonin-Like and Antiserotonin Properties of Psilocybin and Psilocin. Science 136:777-778, 1962.

645. Maxwell, G. M., et al. The Effect of Psilocybin upon the Systemic, Pulmonary and Coronary Circulation of the Intact Dog. Arch. int. Pharmacodyn. 137:108-115, 1962.

646. Castillo, J. C., et al. A Pharmacological Study of N-Methyl-N'-(4-Chlorobenzhydryl) Piperazine Dihydrochloride—a New Antihistamine. J. Pharmacol. exp. Ther. 96: 388-395, 1949.

647. Halpern, B. N. and M. Briot. Comparison of the Acute Toxicity of Several Synthetic Antihistaminics in the Rat. C. R. Soc. Biol. (Paris) 144:887-890, 1950.

648. Swift, J. G. A Study of Sustained Ionic Release Antihistamine. Arch. int. Pharmacodyn. 124:341-348, 1960.

649. Virno, M., et al. Action of Histamine on the Jugular Venous Pressure and Cerebral Circulation of the Dog. Effects of Antihistaminic Drugs (Pyrilamine and Chlorpheniramine) and a Histamine Liberating Agent (48/80 B. W.). J. Pharmacol. exp. Ther. 118: 63-76, 1956.

650. Binet, D. The Study of Polyuria in Convalescence from Acute Sickness. Rev. med. Suisse rom. 15:329-341, 1885.

651. Gibbs, W. and H. A. Hare. Systematic Investigation of Related Chemicals on Animal Organisms. Arch. f. Physiol. (Leipz.) 1:344-359, 1890.

652. Gatgounis, J. and R. P. Walton. Resorcinol Isomers and Pentylenetetrazol; their Centrally Mediated Sympathetic Circulatory Effects. J. Pharmacol. exp. Ther. 127:363-371, 1959.

653. Yoshi, N., et al. Studies on the Unit Discharge of Brainstem Reticular Formation in the Cat. II. Effect of Catechol, Amphetamine, Nembutal and Megimide. Med. J. Osaka Univ. 11:19-33, 1960.

654. Neisser, A. Clinical and Experimental Findings on the Action of Pyrogallus Acid. Z. klin. Med. 1:88-108, 1880.

655. Wylie, D. W. Augmentation of the Pressor Response to Guanethedine by Inhibition of Catechol-O-Methyltransferase. Nature 189:490-491, 1961.

656. Udenfriend, S., et al. Inhibitors of Norepinephrine Metabolism in vivo. Arch. Biochem. 84:249-251, 1959.

657. Bonsmann, M. R. The Pharmacology of the Quinine Alkaloids. Arch. exp. Path. Pharmakol. 205:129-136, 1948.

658. Kirchmann, L. L. Detoxification of Quinidine by Synephrine. Arch. exp. Path. Pharmakol. 192:639-644, 1939.

659. Scott, C. C., et al. Comparison of the Pharmacologic Action of Quinidine and Dihydroquinidine. J. Pharmacol. exp. Ther. 84:184-188, 1945.

660. Cole, J. and D. Dearnaley. Contrasting Tail and other Responses to Morphine and Reserpine in Rats and Mice. Experientia (Basel) 16:78-80, 1960.

661. Brodie, B. B. and P. A. Shore. A Concept for a Role of Serotonin and Norepinephrine as Chemical Mediators in the Brain. Ann. N. Y. Acad. Sci. 66:631-642, 1957.

662. Burn, J. H. and D. B. McDougal, Jr. The Effect of Reserpine on Gangrene Produced by Thiopental in the Mouse Tail. J. Pharmacol. exp. Ther. 131:167-170, 1961.

663. Paasonen, M. K. and O. Krayer. Effect of Reserpine upon the Mammalian Heart. Fed. Proc. 16:326-327, 1957.

664. Canal, N. and A. Maffei-Faccioli. Reversal of the Reserpine-Induced Depletion of Brain Serotonin by a Monoamine Oxidase Inhibitor. J. Neurochem. 5:99-100, 1959.

665. Muscholl, E., and M. Vogt. The Action of Reserpine on the Peripheral Sympathetic System. J. Physiol. (Lond.) 141:132-155, 1958.

666. Sheppard, H. and J. H. Zimmerman. Reserpine and the Levels of Serotonin and Norepinephrine in the Brain. Nature 185:40-41, 1960.

667. Shore, P. A., et al. Release of Brain Norepinephrine by Reserpine. Fed. Proc. 16:335-336, 1957.

668. Wilson, C. W. M., et al. The Effects of Reserpine on Uptake of Epinephrine in Brain and Certain Areas Outside the Blood-Brain Barrier. J. Pharmacol. exp. Ther. 135:11-16, 1961.

669. Trendelenburg, U. and J. S. Gravenstein. Effect of Reserpine Pretreatment on Stimulation of the Accelerans Nerve of the Dog. Science 128:901-902, 1958.

670. Brady, J. V. Animal Experimental Evaluation of Drug Effects upon Behavior. Fed. Proc. 17:1031-1043, 1958.

671. Weiskrantz, L. and W. A. Wilson, Jr. The Effects of Reserpine on Emotional Behavior of Normal and Brain-Operated Monkeys. Ann. N. Y. Acad. Sci. 61:36-55, 1955.

672. Tui, C. and C. Debruille. The Comparative Toxicity and Effectiveness of Scopolamine Hydrobromide ($C_{17}H_{21}O_4N \cdot HBr$) and Scopolamine Aminoxide Hydrobromide ($C_{17}H_{21}O_5N \cdot HBr$). Am. J. Pharm. 117:319-326, 1945.

673. Frommel, E., et al. On the Pharmacodynamic Action of a New Tranquilizer: Methaminodiazepoxide, or Librium. An Experimental Study. Thérapie 15:1233-1244, 1960.

674. Gruhzit, O. M. and A. W. Dox. A Pharmacologic Study of Certain Thiobarbiturates. J. Pharmacol. exp. Ther. 60:125-142, 1937.

675. Silvestrini, B., et al. Action of Synchronizing and Desynchronizing Drugs on Strychnine Induced Convulsive Cortical Activity. Fed. Proc. 16:336, 1957.

676. Costa, E. and G. Zetler. Interactions between Epinephrine and Psychotomimetic Drugs on Cat Nictitating Membrane. Fed. Proc. 17:360, 1958.

677. Winter, D. and M. Timar. Experimental Studies on the Rehypnosis of Animals Just Awakened from Barbiturate Anesthesia. Pharmazie 17:454-455, 1962.

678. Revzin, A. M. and E. Costa. Effects of Exogenous Serotonin on Paleocortical Excitability. Am. J. Physiol. 198:959-961, 1960.

679. Zilberstein, R. Effects of Reserpine, Serotonin and Vasopressin on the Survival of Cold-Stressed Rats. Nature 185:249, 1960.

680. Soulairac, A. and M. L. Soulairac. Action of Reserpine, Serotonin and Iproniazid on the Feeding Behavior of the Rat. C. R. Soc. Biol. (Paris) 154:510-513, 1960.

681. Laroche, M. J. and B. B. Brodie. Lack of Relationship between Inhibition of Monoamine Oxidase and Potentiation of Hexobarbital Hypnosis. J. Pharmacol. exp. Ther. 130:134-137, 1960.

682. Smith, P. K. and W. E. Hambourger. Antipyretic and Toxic Effects of Combinations of Acetanilid with Sodium Bromide and with Caffein. J. Pharmacol. exp. Ther. 55:200-205, 1935.

683. Roholm, K. Fluorine and Fluorine Compounds. Heffter's Hdb. E. 7:1-62, 1938.

684. Muehlberger, C. W. Toxicity Studies of Fluorine Insecticides. J. Pharmacol. exp. Ther. 39:246-248, 1930.

685. Lehman, A. J. Chemicals in Food: A Report to the Association of Food and Drug Officials on Current Developments. Assoc. Food & Drug Officials U. S. Quart. Bull. 15: 122-133, 1951.

686. Ambard, L. and M. S. Trautmann. Demonstration of the Existence of Different Invertases. C. R. Soc. Biol. (Paris) 125:133-135, 1937.

687. Leake, C. D. The Toxicity of Sodium Fluoride in Intravenous Injection in Rabbits. J. Pharmacol. exp. Ther. 33:279-280, 1928.

688. Becker, T., et al. A Theory of Chlorate Poisoning. Arch. exp. Path. Pharmakol. 201: 197-209, 1943.

689. Oltman, T. V. and L. A. Crandal, Jr. The Acute Toxicity of Glyceryl Trinitrate and Sodium Nitrite in Rabbits. J. Pharmacol. exp. Ther. 41:121-126, 1931.

690. Hesse, E. Detoxification of Nitrites. Arch. exp. Path. Pharmakol. 126:209-221, 1927.

691. Dossin, F. Contribution to the Experimental Study of Hypotensive Medication. Arch. int. Pharmacodyn. 21:425-465, 1911.

692. Zipf, H. F. and G. Triller. α-Isoparteine and α-Didehydrosparteine. Arch. exp. Path. Pharmakol. 200:536-550, 1943.

693. Lu, G. Sparteine on Mammalian Circulations. Arch. int. Pharmacodyn. 89:209-222, 1963.

694. Lu, G. Dual Vasomotor Actions of Sparteine. Arch. int. Pharmacodyn. 89:129-144, 1952.

695. Amann, A., et al. A Comparative Study of Strychnine and Strychnine Derivatives. Arch. exp. Path. Pharmakol. 201:161-171, 1943.

696. Ward, J. C. and D. G. Crabtree. Strychnine X. Comparative Accuracies of Stomach Tube and Intraperitoneal Injection Methods of Bioassay. J. Amer. pharm. Ass., sci. Ed. 31: 113-115, 1942.

697. Poe, C. F., et al. Toxicity of Strychnine for Male and Female Rats of Different Ages. J. Pharmacol. exp. Ther. 58:239-242, 1936.

698. Leroy, J. G. and A. F. de Schaepdryver. Catecholamine Levels of Brain and Heart in Mice after Iproniazid Syrosingopine and 10-Methoxydeserpidine. Arch. int. Pharmacodyn. 130:231-234, 1961.

699. Garattini, S., et al. Reserpine Derivatives with Specific Hypotensive or Sedative Activity. Nature (Lond.) 183:1273-1274, 1959.

700. Orlans, F. G. H., et al. Pharmacological Consequences of the Selective Release of Peripheral Norepinephrine by Syrosingopine (SU 3119). J. Pharmacol. exp. Ther. 128: 131-139, 1960.

701. Cook, L. and E. Weidley. Effects of a Series of Psychopharmacological Agents on Isolated Induced Attack Behavior in Mice. Fed. Proc. 19:22, 1960.

702. Heise, G. A. Behavioral Analysis of Tetrabenazine in Animals. Dis. nerv. Syst. 21: (Suppl.) 111-114, 1960.

703. Pletscher, A. Release of 5-Hydroxytryptamine by Benzoquinolizine Derivatives with Sedative Action. Science 126:507, 1957.

704. Astrom, A. and N. H. Persson. The Toxicity of Some Local Anesthetics after Application on Different Mucous Membranes and its Relation to Anesthetic Action on the Nasal Mucosa of the Rabbit. J. Pharmacol. exp. Ther. 132:87-90, 1961.

705. Eichholtz, F. and G. Hoppe. The Convulsive Action of Local Anesthetics and the Effect of Mineral Salts and Adrenaline. Arch. exp. Path. Pharmakol. 173:687-696, 1933.

706. Randall, L. O., et al. The Ganglionic Blocking Action of Thiophanium Derivatives. J. Pharmacol. exp. Ther. 97:48-59, 1949.

707. Hunt, R. and R. R. Renshaw. On Some Effects of Arsonium, Stibonium, Phosphonium and Sulfonium Compounds on the Autonomic Nervous System. J. Pharmacol. exp. Ther. 25:315-355, 1925.

708. Acheson, G. H. and G. K. Moe. The Action of Tetraethylammonium Ion on the Mammalian Circulation. J. Pharmacol. exp. Ther. 87: 220-236, 1946.

709. Acheson, G. H. and G. K. Moe. Some Effects of Tetraethyl Ammonium on the Mammalian Heart. J. Pharmacol. exp. Ther. 84:189-195, 1945.

710. Jodlbauer, A. The Action of Tetramethylammonium Chloride. Arch. int. Pharmacodyn. 7:183-202, 1900.

711. Kuhn, W. L. and E. F. Van Maanen. Effects of Thalidomide on Central Nervous System Drugs. Fed. Proc. 19:264, 1960.

712. Martindale, K., et al. The Effect of Thalidomide in Experimental Gastric Ulcers. J. Pharm. and Pharmacol. 12:153T-158T, 1960.

713. Robinson, M. H. The Effect of Different Intravenous Injection Rates upon the AD_{50}, LD_{50} and Anesthetic Duration of Pentothal in Mice, and Strength-Duration Curves of Depression. J. Pharmacol. exp. Ther. 85: 176-191, 1945.

714. Carmichael, E. B. The Median Lethal Dose (LD_{50}) of Pentothal Sodium for Both Young and Old Guinea Pigs and Rats. Anesthesiology 8:589-593, 1947.

715. Hart, R. The Toxicity and Analgetic Potency of Salicylamide and Certain of its Derivatives as Compared with Established Analgetic-Antipyretic Drugs. J. Pharmacol. exp. Ther. 89:205-209, 1947.

716. Irwin, R. L., et al. The Activity of Certain Lycoramine Derivatives on Muscle. J. Pharmacol. exp. Ther. 134:53-59, 1961.

717. Somjen, G. G. and M. Gill. The Mechanism of the Blockade of Synaptic Transmission in the Mammalian Spinal Cord by Diethyl Ether and by Thiopental. J. Pharmacol. exp. Ther. 140:19-30, 1963.

718. Hey, P. and G. L. Willey. Choline 2: 6-Xylyl Ether Bromide; an Active Quaternary Local Anesthetic. Brit. J. Pharmacol. 9: 471-475, 1954.

719. Nasmyth, P. A. and W. H. H. Andrews. The Antagonism of Cocaine to the Action of Choline 2, 6-Xylyl Ether Bromide at Sympathetic Nerve Endings. Brit. J. Pharmacol. 14:477-483, 1959.

720. McLean, R. A., et al. A Series of 2,6-Disubstituted Phenoxylethyl Ammonium Bromides with True Sympathomimetic Properties. J. Pharmacol. exp. Ther. 129:11-16, 1960.

721. Coupland, R. E. and K. A. Exley. Effects of Choline 2:6 Xylyl Ether Bromide upon the Suprarenal Medulla of the Rat. Brit. J. Pharmacol. 12:306-311, 1957.

722. McLean, R. A., et al. Pharmacology of Trimethyl (2-(2, 6-Dimethylphenoxy) Propyl)-Trimethylammonium Chloride, Monohydrate; Compound 6890 or β-TM10. J. Pharmacol. exp. Ther. 129:17-23, 1960.

723. Everett, G. M., et al. Tremor Induced by Tremorine and its Antagonism by Anti-Parkinson Drugs. Science 124:79, 1956.

724. Everett, G. M., et al. Production of Tremor and a Parkinson-Like Syndrome by 1-4 Dipyrrolidino-2-Butyne, "Tremorine." Fed. Proc. 15:420-421, 1956.

725. Kaelber, W. W. and R. E. Correll. Cortical and Subcortical Electrical Effects of Psychopharmacologic and Tremor-Producing Compounds. Arch. Neurol. Psychiat. (Chic.) 80:544-553, 1958.

726. Korol, B. and L. Soffer. Cardiovascular Activity of D- and L-Octopamine. Pharmacologist 5:247, 1963.

727. Barlow, O. W. Reactions of the Rat to Avertin Crystals, Avertin Fluid and Amylene Hydrate. Arch. Surg. 26:689-695, 1933.

728. Burtner, R. R. and G. Lehmann. The Hypnotic Properties of Some Derivatives of Trihalogenated Alcohols. J. Pharmacol. exp. Ther. 63:183-192, 1938.

729. Barnes, T. C. Relationship of Chemical Structure to Central Nervous System Effects of Tranquilizing and Anticonvulsant Drugs. J. Amer. pharm. Ass., sci. Ed. 49:415-417, 1960.

730. Tedeschi, D. H., et al. The Neuropharmacology of Trifluoperazine: a Potent Psychotherapeutic Agent. Arch. int. Pharmacodyn. 122:129-143, 1957.

731. Richards, R. K. and G. M. Everett. Tridione: A New Anticonvulsant Drug. J. Lab. clin. Med. 31:1330-1336, 1946.

732. Hoppe, J. O. and A. M. Lands. The Toxicologic Properties of N, N-Dimethyl-N'(3-Thenyl-N' (2-Pyridyl) Ethylenediamine Hydrochloride (Thenfadil): A New Antihistamine Drug. J. Pharmacol. exp. Ther. 97:371-378, 1949.

733. Macri, F. V. Curare-Like Activity of Some Bis-Fluorenyl-Bis-Quaternary Ammonium Compounds. Proc. Soc. exp. Biol. (N.Y.) 85: 603-606, 1954.

734. Berger, F. M. and R. P. Schwartz. The Toxicity and Muscular Effect of d-Tubocurarine Combined with β-Erythroidine, Myanesin or Evipal. J. Pharmacol. exp. Ther. 93:362-367, 1948.

735. Marsh, D. F. and M. H. Pelletier. Curariform Activity of Quaternary Ammonium Iodides Derived from Cinchona Alkaloids. J. Pharmacol. exp. Ther. 92:127-130, 1948.

736. Everett, G. M. Pharmacological Studies of d-Tubocurarine and Other Curare Fractions. J. Pharmacol. exp. Ther. 92:236-248, 1948.

737. Barbour, H. G. and L. L. Maurer. Tyramine as a Morphine Antagonist. J. Pharmacol. exp. Ther. 15:305-330, 1920.

738. Kuntzman, R. and M. Jacobson. Depletion of Heart Norepinephrine by Tyramine. Pharmacologist 5:258, 1963.

739. Nasmyth, P. A. In: Ciba Foundation Symposium, p. 337, eds. Vane, J. R., et al. Little Brown, Boston, 1960.

740. Egami, M. A Pharmacological Study of Afferent Impulse from the Small Intestine. Jap. J. Pharmacol. 4:160-167, 1955.

741. Barer, G. R. and E. Nusser. Cardiac Output during Excitation of Chemo-Reflexes in the Cat. Brit. J. Pharmacol. 13:372-377, 1958.

742. Benforado, J. M., et al. Studies on Veratrum Alkaloids. XXIX. The Action of Some Germine Esters and of Veratridine upon Blood Pressure, Heart Rate and Femoral Blood Flow in the Dog. J. Pharmacol. exp. Ther. 130:311-320, 1960.

743. Hagen, E. C. and J. L. Radomski. The Toxicity of 3-(Acetonylbenzyl)-4-Hydroxycoumarin (Warfarin) to Laboratory Animals. J. Am. pharm. Ass. 42:379-382, 1953.

744. Preziosi, P., et al. On the Pulmonary and Cardiovascular Effects of Warfarin Sodium. Arch. int. Pharmacodyn. 123:227-238, 1959.

745. Röthlin, E. and R. Hamet. On the Toxicity and Adrenolytic Activity of Pseudocorynathine Compared with That of Corynanthine and Yohimbine. Arch. int. Pharmacodyn. 50:241-250, 1935.

746. Barrett, E., et al. A Comparison of the Activity of Various Adrenolytic Agents in Antagonizing the Epinephrine Potentiation Induced by Ganglionic Blockage. J. Pharmacol. exp. Ther. 110:3-4, 1954.

747. McCubbin, J. W. and I. Page. Do Ganglionic Blocking Agents and Reserpine Affect Central Vasomotor Activity? Circ. Res. 6:816-824, 1958.

748. Nasmyth, P. A. An Investigation of the Action of Tyramine and its Interrelationship with the Effects of Other Sympathomimetic Amines. Brit. J. Pharmacol. 18:65-75, 1962.

749. György, L. and M. Dóda. Adrenaline Tachyphylaxis after Dibenamine. Arch. int. Pharmacodyn. 124:66-75, 1960.

750. Riker, W. K. and A. Komalahiranya. Observations on the Frequency Dependence of Sympathetic Ganglionic Blockade. J. Pharmacol. exp. Ther. 137:267-274, 1962.

751. Melville, K. I. Studies on the Cardiovascular Actions of Chlorpromazine. I. Antiadrenergic and Antifibrillatory Actions. Arch. int. Pharmacodyn. 115:278-305, 1958.

752. Ross, J., Jr., et al. The Influence of Intra-cardiac Baroreceptors on Venous Return, Systemic Vascular Volume and Peripheral Resistance. J. Clin. Inves, 40:563-572, 1961.

753. Byck, R. The Effect of C_6 on the Carotid Chemoreceptor Response to Nicotine and Cyanide. Brit. J. Pharmacol. 16:15-22, 1961.

754. Lamond, D. R. and C. W. Emmens. The Effect of Hypophysectomy on the Mouse Uterine Response to Gonadotrophins. J. Endocrin. 18:251-261, 1959.

755. Boccabella, A. V. Reinitiation and Restoration of Spermatogenesis with Testosterone Propionate and Other Hormones after a Long-Term Post-hypophysectomy Regression Period. Endocrinology 72:787-798, 1963.

756. Smith, B. D. and J. T. Bradburg. Ovarian Weight Response to Varying Doses of Estrogens in Intact and Hypophysectomized Rats. Proc. Sec. exp. Biol. (N.Y.) 107:946-949, 1961.

757. Fain, J. N. and A. E. Wilhelmi. Effects of Adrenalectomy, Hypophysectomy, Growth Hormone and Thyroxine on Fatty Acid Synthesis in vivo. Endocrinology 71:541-548, 1962.

758. Nejad, N. S., et al. Hormonal Repair of Defective Lipogenesis from Glucose in the Liver of the Hypophysectomized Rat. Endocrinology 71:107-112, 1962.

759. Meineke, H. A. and R. C. Crafts. Correlation Between Oxygen Consumption and Erythropoiesis in Hypophysectomized Rats Treated with Various Doses of Thyroxine. Proc. Soc. exp. Biol. (N.Y.) 102:121-124, 1959.

760. Evans, E. S., et al. Erythropoietic Response to Calorigenic Hormones. Endocrinology 68:517-532, 1961.

761. Baker, B. L. Elevation of Proteolytic Activity in the Pancreas of Hypophysectomized Rats by Hormonal Therapy. Proc. Soc. Biol. (N.Y.) 108:238-242, 1961.

762. De Bodo, R. C. and M. W. Sinkoff. The Role of Growth Hormone in Carbohydrate Metabolism. Ann. N. Y. Acad. Sci. 57:23-60, 1953.

763. Wick, A. N., et al. Effect of 11-Desoxy-corticosterone Acetate upon Carbohydrate Utilization by the Depancreated Rat. Proc. Soc. exp. Biol. (N.Y.) 71:445-446, 1949.

764. Scow, R. O., et al. Effect of Hypophysectomy on the Insulin Requirement and Response to Fasting of "Totally" Pancreatectomized Rats. Endocrinology 61:380-391, 1957.

765. Allegretti, N. Gamma-Globulin Concentration in Normal and Depancreatized Rats Subjected to Formalin Stress. Arch. int. Pharmacodyn. 93:367-372, 1953.

766. Ingle, D. J., et al. Comparison of the Effect of 11-ketoprogesterone, 11α-Hydroxyprogesterone and 11β-Hydroxyprogesterone upon the Glycosuria of the Partially Depancreatized Rat. Endocrinology 53:221-225, 1953.

767. Ingle, D. J. Effect of 11-Desoxycorticosterone Acetate on the Glycosuria of Partially Depancreatized Rats. Proc. Soc. exp. Biol. (N.Y.) 69:329-330, 1948.

768. Greeley, P. O. The Action of Insulin as Indicated by Depancreatized Herbivora. Am. J. Physiol. 150:46-51, 1947.

769. Gastaldi, F. Glycemic Changes Caused by Testosterone Propionate in Normal and Pancreatectomized Dogs. Studi Sassaresi 25:601-606, 1947.

770. Gillman, J. The Relationship of Hyperglycemia to Hyperlipemia and Ketonaemia in Depancreatized Baboons (Papio Ursinus). J. Endocrin. 17:349-362, 1958.

771. Glasser, S. R. and J. L. Izzo. The Influence of Adrenalectomy on the Metabolic Actions of Glucogon in the Fasting Rat. Endocrinology 70:54-61, 1962.

772. Gross, F. and P. Lichtlen. Experimental Renal Hypertension: Renal Content of Kidneys in Intact and Adrenalectomized Rats Given Cortexone. Am. J. Physiol. 195:543-548, 1958.

773. Smith, S., et al. Some Metabolic Effects of Diethylstilbestrol and Deoxycorticosterone Acetate in Adrenalectomized and Intact Male Rats. Proc. West. Va. Acad. Sci. 32:22-25, 1960.

774. Pores, G. Effects of Aldosterone on Carbohydrate Metabolism of Normal and Adrenalectomized Rats. C. R. Soc. Biol. (Paris) 155:790-792, 1961.

775. Hungerford, G. F. Effect of Adrenalectomy and Hydrocortisone on Lymph Glucose in Rats. Proc. Soc. exp. Biol. (N.Y.) 100:754-756, 1959.

776. Pederson-Bjergaard, K. and M. Tonnesen. The Effects of Steroid Hormones on Muscular Activity in Rats. Acta endocrinal 17: 329-337, 1954.

777. Aterman, K. Cortisol and Spermiogenesis. Acta endocrinal 22:371-378, 1956.

778. Fain, J. N. Effects of Dexamethasone and Growth Hormone on Fatty Acid Mobilization and Glucose Utilization in Adrenalectomized Rats. Endocrinology 71:633-635, 1962.

779. Peres, G. and G. Zwingelstein. Action of Aldosterone on the Blood Proteins of the Normal and Adrenalectomized Rat. J. physiol. (Paris) 53:444-446, 1961.

780. Peters, G. Distribution of Water and Electrolytes in the Organism in Normal and Adrenalectomized, Untreated Rats or Such Rats Treated with Adrenocortical Hormone, and the Influence of Large Oral Water Loads. Arch. exp. Pathol. Pharmakol. 237:119-150, 1959.

781. Winter, H., et al. Antibody Formation in the Adrenalectomized Rat and the Effect of Cortisone. Inter. Arch. Allergy Appl. Immunol. 19:360-376, 1961.

782. Kahlson, G. and S. Renvall. Atrophy of Salivary Gland Following Adrenalectomy or Hypophysectomy and the Effect of Deoxycorticosterone in Cats. Acta physiol. scand. 37: 150-158, 1956.

783. Sesso, A. and R. Migliorini. Nucleic Acid Content and Amylase Activity in the Pancreas of the Rat Following Adrenalectomy and Cortisone Administration. Acta physiol. lat.-amer. 9:5-12, 1959.

784. Gross, F. and H. Haefeli. The Activity of Deoxycorticosterone, Cortisone, and Antihistamine Substances on the Anaphylactic Shock of Adrenalectomized Guinea Pigs. Intern. Arch. Allergy Appl. Immunol. 3:44-53, 1952.

785. Berlin, R. D., et al. Abrupt Changes of Water and Sodium Excretion in Normal and Adrenalectomized Dogs. Am. J. Physiol. 199:275-280, 1960.

786. Daane, T. A. and W. R. Lyons. Effect of Estrone, Progesterone, and Pituitary Mammotropin on the Mammary Glands of Castrated C_3H Male Mice. Endocrinology 55: 191-199, 1954.

787. Kitay, J. T. Pituitary-Adrenal Function in the Rat after Gonadectomy and Gonadol Hormone Replacement. Endocrinology 73:253-260, 1963.

788. Meli, A. Route of Administration as a Factor Influencing the Biological Activity of Certain Androgens and their Corresponding 3-Cyclopentyl Enol Ethers. Endocrinology 72: 715-719, 1963.

789. Rudolph, G. G. and W. R. Starnes. Effect of Castration and Testosterone Administration on Seminal Vesicles and Prostates of Rats. Am. J. Physiol. 179:415-418, 1954.

790. Mandel, P., et al. Effect of Testosterone on the Calcium Balance in the Rat. C. R. Acad. Sci. (Paris) 148:713-715, 1954.

791. Kanai, T. Effect of Androgen on Fine Structure of the Prostate of Castrated Rats. II. The Effect of Administration of Small Doses of Testosterone 3 Days After Castration. Tohoku J. Exptl. Med. 75:309-318, 1961.

792. Levey, H. A. and C. M. Szego. Effects of Castration and Androgen Administration on Metabolic Characteristics of the Guinea Pig Seminal Vesicle. Am. J. Physiol. 183:371-376, 1955.

793. Dagradi, A. and G. Peronato. Influence of the Gonads on Carbohydrate Metabolism. Patol. sper. chir. 1:420-429, 1953.

794. Grunt, J. A. Exogenous Androgen and Nondirected Hyperexcitability in Castrated Male Guinea Pigs. Proc. Soc. exp. Biol. (N. Y.) 85: 540-542, 1954.

795. Munford, R. E. The Effect of Cortisol Acetate on Estrone-Induced Mammary Gland Growth in Immature Ovariectomized Albino Mice. J. Endocrin. 16:72-79, 1957.

796. Grosvenor, C. E. Effects of Estrogen upon Thyroidal I^{131} Release and Excretion of Thyroxine in Ovariectomized Rats. Endocrinology 70:673-678, 1962.

797. Lerner, J., et al. Pregnancy Maintenance in Ovariectomized Rats with 16α, 17α Dihydroxyprogesterone Derivatives and Other Progestogens. Endocrinology 70:283-287, 1962.

798. Woolley, D. E. and P. S. Timiras. The Gonad-Brain Relationship: Effects of Female

Sex Hormones on Electroshock Convulsions in the Rat. Endocrinology 72:196-209, 1963.

799. Escobar del Rey, F. and G. Morreale de Escobar. Studies on the Peripheral Disappearance of Thyroid Hormone. Acta endocrin. 29:161-175, 1958.

800. Barker, S. B., et al. Metabolic Effects of Thyroxine Injected into Normal, Thiouracil-Treated, and Thyroidectomized Rats. Endocrinology 45:624-627, 1949.

801. Halmi, N. S., et al. Improved Intravenous Glucose Tolerance in Thyroidectomized or Hypophysectomized Rats Treated with Triiodothyronine. Endocrinology 64:618-621, 1959.

802. De Bastiani, G., et al. Significance of the Thyrotropic Hormone of the Hypophysis in the Syndrome Resulting from Thyroidectomy. Boll. soc. ital. biol. sper. 32:200-204, 1956.

803. Von Berswordt-Wallrabe, R. and C. W. Turner. Successful Replacement Therapy in Lactating Thyro-parathyroidectomized Rats. Proc. soc. exp. Biol. (N.Y.) 104:113-116, 1960.

804. Harrison, R. G., and T. J. Barnett. Production of Arthritis in Thyroparathyroidectomized Rat by Injections of Deoxycorticosterone Acetate. Ann. rheum. Dis. 12:275-282, 1953.

805. Cramer, C. F. Participation of Parathyroid Glands in Control of Calcium Absorption in Dogs. Endocrinology 72:192-196, 1963.

806. Gordon, A. H. The Parathyroid Hormone. Congr. intern. biochim., Resumes communs, 2e Congr. Paris:53-54, 1952.

807. Talmage, R. V., et al. Effect of Parathyroid Extract and Phosphate Salts on Renal Calcium and Phosphate Excretion after Parathyroidectomy. Proc. soc. exp. Biol. (N.Y.) 88:600-604, 1955.

808. Laron, Z., et al. Phosphaturic Effect of Cortisone in Normal and Parathyroidectomized Rats. Proc. soc. exp. Biol. (N.Y.) 96:649-651, 1957.

809. Page, I. H. and J. W. McCubbin. Effect of Pentobarbital and Atropine on Arterial Pressure Response to Ganglion Blocking Agents. Am. J. Physiol. 194:597-600, 1958.

810. Costa, E., et al. Interactions between Reserpine, Chlorpromazine, and Imipramine. Experientia (Basel) 16:461-463, 1960.

811. Crout, J. R. Inhibition of Catechol-O-Methyl Transferase by Pyrogallol in the Rat. Biochem. Pharmacol. 6:47-50, 1961.

812. Finkleman, B. On the Nature of Inhibition in the Intestines. J. Physiol. (Lond.) 70:145-157, 1930.

813. Chorover, S. L. Effects of Mescaline and Chlorpromazine on Two Aspects of Locomotor Activity in Rats. Fed. Proc. 19:22, 1960.

814. Freyburger, W. A., et al. The Pharmacology of 5-Hydroxytryptamine (Serotonin). J. Pharmacol. exp. Ther. 105:80-86, 1952.

815. Gutman, J. and M. Chaimovitz. The Effect of Anesthetics on Blood Pressure Response to Pain. Arch. int. Pharmacodyn. 137:40-48. 1962.

816. Millar, R. A., et al. Plasma, Adrenaline and Noradrenaline after Phenoxybenzamine Administration, and During Haemorrhagic Hypotension, in Normal and Adrenalectomized Dogs. Brit. J. Pharmacol. 14:9-13, 1959.

817. Walker, H. A., et al. The Effect of 1-Hydrazinophthalazine (C-5968) and Related Compounds on the Cardiovascular System of Dogs. J. Pharmacol. exp. Ther. 101:368-378, 1951.

818. Haury, V. G. and M. E. Drake. The Effect of Intravenous Injections of Sodium Diphenyl Hydantoinate (Dilantin) on Respiration, Blood Pressure, and the Vagus Nerve. J. Pharmacol. exp. Ther. 68:36-40, 1940.

819. Drake, M. E., V. G. Haury, and C. M. Gruber: The Action of Sodium Diphenyl Hydantoinate (Dilantin) on the Excised and Intact Uterus. Arch. int. Pharmacodyn. 43:288-291, 1939.

820. Belenky, M. L. and M. Vitolina. The pharmacological analysis of the hyperthermia caused by phenamine (amphetamine). Int. J. Neuropharmacol. 1:1-7, 1962.

821. Benfey, B. G. and D. R. Varma. Studies on the cardiovascular actions of antisympathomimetic drugs. Int. J. Neuropharmacol. 1:9-12, 1962.

822. Campos, H. A. and F. E. Shideman. Subcellular distribution of catecholamines in the dog heart. Int. J. Neuropharmacol. 1:13-22, 1962.

823. Kido, R. and K. Yamamoto. An analysis of tranquilizers in chronically electrode implanted cat. Int. J. Neuropharmacol. 1:49-53, 1962.

824. White, R. P. and E. J. Westerbeke. Relationship between central anticholinergic actions and antiparkinson efficacy of phenothiazine derivatives. Int. J. Neuropharmacol. 1:213-216, 1962.

825. Knapp, D. E. and E. F. Domino. Action of nicotine on the ascending reticular activating system. Int. J. Neuropharmacol. 1:333-351, 1962.

826. Riehl, J. L., et al. Comparison of the effects of arecoline and muscarine on the central nervous system. Int. J. Neuropharmacol. 1:393-401, 1962.

827. Knapp, D. E. and E. F. Domino. Species differences in the EEG response to epinephrine, 5-hydroxytryptamine and nicotine in brainstem transected animals. Int. J. Neuropharmacol. 2:51-55, 1963.

828. Koll, W., et al. The predilective action of small doses of morphine on nociceptive spinal reflexes of low spinal cats. Int. J. Neuropharmacol. 2:57-65, 1963.

829. Liberson, W. I., et al. Effects of chlorodiazepoxide (Librium) on fixated behavior in rats. Int. J. Neuropharmacol. 2:67-78, 1963.

830. Spector, S., et al. Association of behavioral effects of pargyline, a non-hydrazide MAO inhibitor with increase in brain norepinephrine. Int. J. Neuropharmacol. 2:81-93, 1963.

831. Herz, A. Excitation and inhibition of cholinoceptive brain structures and its relationship to pharmacological induced behavior changes. Int. J. Neuropharmacol. 2:205-216, 1963.

832. White, R. P. and C. B. Nash. Catechol antagonism to the EEG effects of reserpine, chlorpromazine, pentobarbital and atropine. Int. J. Neuropharmacol. 2:249-254, 1963.

833. Liberson, W. T., et al. Synaptic transmission in the hippocampus and psychopharmacological agents. Int. J. Neuropharmacol. 2:291-302, 1964.

834. Olds, M. E. and J. Olds. Pharmacological patterns in subcortical reinforcement behavior. Int. J. Neuropharmacol. 2:309-325, 1964.

835. Steiner, W. G., et al. An electroencephalographic study of some structural aspects of d-amphetamine antagonism in phenothiazine and related compounds. Int. J. Neuropharmacol. 2:327-335, 1964.

836. Sigg, E. B. and T. D. Sigg. Sympathetic stimulation and blockade of the urinary bladder in cat. Int. J. Neuropharmacol. 3:241-251, 1964.

837. Stille, G. and A. Sayers. The effect of antidepressant drugs on the convulsive excitability of brain structures. Int. J. Neuropharmacol. 3:605-609, 1964.

838. Metysova, J. and J. Metys. Pharmacological properties of the desmethyl derivatives of some antidepressants of imipramine type. Int. J. Neuropharmacol. 4:111-124, 1965.

839. Herz, A., et al. The importance of lipid-solubility for the central action of cholinolytic drugs. Int. J. Neuropharmacol 4:207-218, 1965.

840. Dungan, K. M., et al. Amidephrine - I: Pharmacologic characterization of a sympathomimetic alkylsulfonamidophenethanolamine. Int. J. Neuropharmacol. 4:219-234, 1965.

841. Jurna, I. Depression of facilitatory influences on spinal motor activity by carisoprodol. Int. J. Neuropharmacol. 4:245-254, 1965.

842. Eidelberg, E., et al. Spectrum analysis of EEG changes induced by psychotomimetic agents. Int. J. Neuropharmacol. 4:255-264, 1965.

843. Schalleck, W., et al. Effects of mogadon on responses to stimulation of sciatic nerve, amygdala and hypothalamus of cat. Int. J. Neuropharmacol. 4:317-326, 1965.

844. Stille, G., et al. The pharmacological properties of a potent neurotropic compound from the dibenzothiazepine group. Int. J. Neuropharmacol. 4:375-391, 1965.

845. Diamantis, W. and M. Kletzkin. Evaluation of muscle relaxant drugs by head-drop and by decerebrate rigidity. Int. J. Neuropharmacol. 5:305-310, 1966.

846. Straw, R. N. and C. L. Mitchell. Effect of phenobarbital on cortical afterdischarge and overt seizure patterns in the cat. Int. J. Neuropharmacol. 5:323-330, 1966.

847. Jurna, I. Depression of the dorsal root potential of the cat spinal cord by amidopyrine. Int. J. Neuropharmacol. 5:361-365, 1966.

848. Horovitz, Z. P., et al. Effects of drugs on the mouse-killing (muricide) test and its relationship to amygdaloid function. Int. J. Neuropharmacol. 5:405-411, 1966.

849. McClane, T. K. and W. R. Martin. Effects of morphine, nalorphine, cyclazocine, and naloxone on the flexor reflex. Int. J. Neuropharmacol. 6:89-98, 1967.

850. Brimblecombe, R. W. and D. M. Green. Central effects of imipramine-like antidepressants in relation to their peripheral anticholinergic activity. Int. J. Neuropharmacol. 6:133-142, 1967.

851. Stille, G. and A. Sayers. Motor convulsions and EEG during maximal electroshock in the rat. Int. J. Neuropharmacol. 6:169-174, 1967.

852. Bohdanecky, Z., and M. E. Jarvik. Impairment of one-trial passive avoidance learning in mice by scopolamine, scopolamine methyl-bromide, and physostigmine. Int. J. Neuropharmacol. 6:217-222, 1967.

853. Norton, S. An analysis of cat behavior using chlorpromazine and amphetamine. Int. J. Neuropharmacol. 6:307-316, 1967.

854. Collins, R. J. and V. R. Simonton. Inhibition of evoked potentials by caudate stimulation and its antagonism by centrally acting drugs. Int. J. Neuropharmacol. 6:349-356, 1967.

855. Cummings, J. R., et al. Cardiovascular actions of guancydine in normotensive and hypertensive animals. J. Pharmacol. Exp. Therap. 161:88-97, 1968.

856. Dilts, S. L. and C. A. Berry. Effect of cholinergic drugs on passive avoidance in the mouse. J. Pharmacol. Exp. Therap. 158:278-285, 1967.

857. King, A. B. and J. A. Thomas. Effect of exogenous dopamine on rat adrenal ascorbic acid. J. Pharmacol. Exp. Therap. 159:18-21, 1968.

858. Lawson, J. W. Antiarrhythmic activity of some isoquinoline derivatives determined by a rapid screening procedure in the mouse. J. Pharmacol. Exp. Therap. 160:22-31, 1968.

859. Schumacher, H., et al. A comparison of the teratogenic activity of thalidomide in rabbits and rats. J. Pharmacol. Exp. Therap. 160:189-200, 1968.

860. Goldberg, S. J., et al. The pulmonary and systemic hemodynamic effects produced by meperidine and hydroxyzine. J. Pharmacol. Exp. Therap. 159:306-313, 1968.

861. Creveling, C. R., et al. The depletion of cardiac norepinephrine by 3,5-dihydroxy-4-methoxyphenethylamine and related compounds. J. Pharmacol. Exp. Therap. 158:46-54, 1967.

862. Lehr, D., et al. Copious drinking and simultaneous inhibition of urine flow elicited by beta-adrenergic stimulation and contrary effect of alpha-adrenergic stimulation. J. Pharmacol. Exp. Therap. 158:150-163, 1967.

863. McChesney, E. W., et al. The hyperglycemic action of some analogs of epinephrine. Soc. Exptl. Biol. Med. 71:220-223, 1949.

864. Pratesi, P., et al. Chemical structure and biologic activity of the catechol amines. I. Influence of the N-alkyl substitution. Farmaco. Ed. Sci. 18:920-931, 1963.

865. McCutcheon, R. S. Canine blood sugar and lactic acid responses to adrenergic amines after adrenergic block. J. Pharmacol. Exp. Therap. 136:209-212, 1962.

866. Mayer, S., et al. The effect of adrenergic blocking agents on some metabolic actions of catecholamines. J. Pharmacol. Exp. Therap. 134:18-27, 1961.

867. Bhagat, B. The influence of sympathetic nervous activity on cardiac catecholamine levels. J. Pharmacol. Exp. Therap. 157:74-80, 1967.

868. Maitre, L. Monoamine oxidase inhibiting properties of SU-11,739 in the rat. Comparison with pargyline, tranylcypromine and iproniazid. J. Pharmacol. Exp. Therap. 157:81-88, 1967.

869. Saito, S. and Y. Tokunaga. Some correlations between picrotoxin-induced seizures and γ-aminobutyric acid in animal brain. J. Pharmacol. Exp. Therap. 157:546-554, 1967.

870. Lorenzo, A. V. and C. F. Barlow. Effect of strychnine convulsions upon the entry of S^{35} sulfate into the cat central nervous system. J. Pharmacol. Exp. Therap. 157:555-564, 1967.

871. Vaillant, G. E. A comparison of antagonists of physostigmine-induced suppression of behavior. J. Pharmacol. Exp. Therap. 157:636-648, 1967.

872. Long, J. P., et al. A pharmacologic evaluation of hemicholinium analogs. J. Pharmacol. Exp. Therap. 155:223-230, 1967.

873. Herman, E. H. and C. D. Barnes. Drug modification of the Schiff-Sherrington phenomenon. J. Pharmacol. Exp. Therap. 156:48-54, 1967.

874. Latz, A., et al. Maze learning after the administration of antidepressant drugs. J. Pharmacol. Exp. Therap. 156:76-84, 1967.

875. Chai, C. Y. and S. C. Wang. Cardiovascular actions of diazepam in the cat. J. Pharmacol. Exp. Therap. 154:271-280, 1966.

876. Oliverio, A. Effects of mecomylamine on avoidance conditioning and maze learning of mice. J. Pharmacol. Exp. Therap. 154:350-356, 1966.

877. Bainbridge, J. G. and D. T. Greenwood. Tranquillizing effects of propranolol demonstrated in rats. Neuropharmacol. 10:453-458, 1971.

878. Suwandi, I. S. and J. A. Bevan. Antagonism of lobeline by ganglion-blocking agents of afferent nerve endings. J. Pharmacol. Exp. Therap. 153:1-7, 1966.

879. Bhagat, B. and J. Gilliam, Jr. Factors influencing the depletion of cardiac norepinephrine by tyramine. J. Pharmacol. Exp. Therap. 153:191-196, 1966.

880. Kulharni, A. S. and F. E. Shideman. Sensitivities of the brains of infant and adult rats to the catecholamine-depleting actions of reserpine and tetrabenazine. J. Pharmacol. Exp. Therap. 153:428-433, 1965.

BIBLIOGRAPHY

881. Swinyard, E. A. and A. W. Castellion. Anticonvulsant properties of some benzodiazephines. J. Pharmacol. Exp. Therap. 151:369-375, 1966.

882. Williams, B., et al. Electrical activity of the prepyriform cortex after reserpine in the rat. J. Pharmacol. Exp. Therap. 150:10-16, 1965.

883. Eble, J. N., and A. Rudzik. The potentiation of the pressor response to tyramine by amphetamine in the anesthetized dog. J. Pharmacol. Exp. Therap. 150:375-381, 1965.

884. Boshart, C. R., et al. The effects of reserpine, guanethidine and other automatic drugs on free fatty acid mobilization induced by phentolamine. J. Pharmacol. Exp. Therap. 149:57-64, 1965.

885. Chen, G., et al. An investigation on the sympathomimetic properties of phencyclidine by comparison with cocaine and desoxyephedrine. J. Pharmacol. Exp. Therap. 149:71-78, 1965.

886. Bircher, R. P., et al. Effects of hexamethonium and tetraethylammonium on cardiac arrhythmias produced by pentylenetetrazol, picrotoxin and deslanoside in dogs. J. Pharmacol. Exp. Therap. 149:91-97, 1965.

887. Lish, P. M., et al. Pharmacological and toxicological properties of two new β-adrenergic receptor antagonists. J. Pharmacol. Exp. Therap. 149:161-173, 1965.

888. Bhagat, B. Pressor responses to amphetamine in the spinal cat and its influence on tachyphylaxis to tyramine. J. Pharmacol. Exp. Therap. 149:206-211, 1965.

889. Norton, S. and R. E. Jewett. Effect of drugs on spontaneous slow potential oscillations of the cerebral cortex. J. Pharmacol. Exp. Therap. 149:301-310, 1965.

890. Gaitonde, B. B., et al. Central emetic action and toxic effects of digitalis in cats. J. Pharmacol. Exp. Therap. 147:409-415, 1965.

891. Straw, R. N. and C. L. Mitchell. The effects of morphine, pentobarbitol, pentazocine and nalorphine on bioelectrical potentials evoked in the brain stem of the cat by electrical stimulation of the tooth pulp. J. Pharmacol. Exp. Therap. 146:7-15, 1964.

892. Rosenberg, F. J. and P. J. Savarie. Histamine and the reversal of chlorpromazine-induced depression. J. Pharmacol. Exp. Therap. 146:180-185, 1964.

893. Lucchesi, B. R. The action of nethalide upon experimentally induced cardiac arrhythmias. J. Pharmacol. Exp. Therap. 145:286-291, 1964.

894. Martin, W. R., et al. Use of hindlimb reflexes of the chronic spinal dog for comparing analgesics. J. Pharmacol. Exp. Therap. 144:8-11, 1964.

895. Weiss, B. and V. G. Laties. Effects of amphetamine, chlorpromazine, pentobarbital, and ethanol on operant response duration. J. Pharmacol. Exp. Therap. 144:17-23, 1964.

896. Swinyard, E. A., et al. Effect of epinephrine and norepinephrine on excitability of central nervous system of mice. J. Pharmacol. Exp. Therap. 144:52-59, 1964.

897. Erij, D. and R. Mendez. The modification of digitalis intoxication by excluding adrenergic influences on the heart. J. Pharmacol. Exp. Therap. 144:97-103, 1964.

898. Nechay, B. R. Potentiation of diuretic effects of methyl xanthines and pyrimidines by carbonic anhydrase inhibitors. J. Pharmacol. Exp. Therap. 144:276-283, 1964.

899. Sulser, F., et al. The action of desmethylimipramine in counteracting sedation and cholinergic effects of reserpine-like drugs. J. Pharmacol. Exp. Therap. 144:321-330, 1964.

900. Esplin, D. W. and B. Zablocka. Pilocarpine blockade of spinal inhibition in cats. J. Pharmacol. Exp. Therap. 143:174-180, 1964.

901. Kirpekar, S. M. and P. Cervoni. Effect of cocaine, phenoxybenzamine and phentolamine on the catecholamine output from spleen and adrenal medulla. J. Pharmacol. Exp. Therap. 142:59-70, 1963.

902. Zimmerman, A. M. and L. S. Harris. Microcirculation effects of guanethidine and reserpine. J. Pharmacol. Exp. Therap. 142:76-82, 1963.

903. Goldberg, M. E., et al. Psychopharmacological effects of reversible cholinesterase inhibition induced by N-methyl 3-isopropyl phenyl carbamate (compound 10854). J. Pharmacol. Exp. Therap. 141:244-252, 1963.

904. Eckhardt, E. T., and F. W. Schweler. The pharmacology of methane sulfonyl choline. J. Pharmacol. Exp. Therap. 141:343-348, 1963.

905. Winter, C. A., et al. Anti-inflammatory and anti-pyretic activities of indomethacin, (1-p-chlorobenzoyl)-5-methozy-2-methyl-indole-3-acetic acid. J. Pharmacol. Exp. Therap. 141:369-376, 1963.

906. Brodey, J. F., et al. An electrographic study of psilocin and 4-methyl-α-methyl tryptamine (MP-809). J. Pharmacol. Exp. Therap. 140:8-18, 1963.

907. Natoff, I. L. Influence of the route of administration on the toxicity of some cholinesterase inhibitors. J. Pharm. Pharmacol. 19:612-616, 1967.

908. Blane, G. F. Blockade of bradykinin-induced nociception in the rat as a test for analgesic drugs with particular reference to morphine antagonists. J. Pharm. Pharmac. 19:367-373, 1967.

909. Brittain, R. T. The pharmacology of 2-amino-4-methyl-6-phenylamino-1,3,5-triazine, a centrally acting muscle relaxant. J. Pharm. Pharmac. 18:294-304, 1966.

910. Ross, S. B. and A. L. Renyi. In vivo inhibition of ³H-noradrenaline uptake by mouse brain slices in vitro. J. Pharm. Pharmac. 18: 322-323, 1966.

911. Buckett, W. R. Some pharmacological studies with 14-cinnamoyloxycodeinone. J. Pharm. Pharmac. 17:759-760, 1965.

912. Korol, B., et al. Some cardiovascular studies on octopamine. Arch. int. Pharmacodyn. 171: 415-424, 1968.

913. Raines, A., et al. The effect of spinal section on ventricular rhythm disorders induced by ouabain. Arch. int. Pharmacodyn. 170: 485-490, 1967.

914. Sergman, F., et al. Action of phentolamine on respiratory reflexes in the rabbit. Arch. int. Pharmacodyn. 169:348-353, 1967.

915. Cohen, M. A comparative study of anti-cholinergic psychotomimetic agents in mice and dogs. Arch. int. Pharmacodyn. 169:412-420, 1967.

916. Stanton, H. C. and C. M. Cooper. Antihypertensive effects of drugs measured in unanesthetized rats with established adrenal regeneration hypertension. Arch. int. Pharmacodyn. 168:1-13, 1967.

917. McKean, W. B., Jr. In vivo antiserotonin activity in the unanesthetized guinea pig. Arch. int. Pharmacodyn. 168:373-382, 1967.

918. Straw, R. N. and C. L. Mitchell. The effect of pentylenetetrazol on biochemical activity recorded from the cat brain. Arch. int. Pharmacodyn. 186:456-466, 1967.

919. Westfall, T. C. Accumulation of norepinephrine in rat tissue following treatment with three β-adrenergic antagonists. Arch. int. Pharmacodyn. 167:69-79, 1967.

920. Banziger, R. and D. Hane. Evaluation of a new convulsant for anticonvulsant screening. Arch. int. Pharmacodyn. 167:245-249, 1967.

921. Uyeno, E. T. Effects of mescaline and psilocybin on dominant behavior of the rat. Arch. int. Pharmacodyn. 166:60-64, 1967.

922. Georges, A., et al. Cardiotonic properties of formiloxin, a semi-synthetic glycoside. Arch. int. Pharmacodyn. 164:47-55, 1966.

923. Coscia, L., et al. A new synthetic analgesic drug, p-phenetidine-α-N-n-propylpropionamide (FC 379). Arch. int. Pharmacodyn. 164:331-339, 1966.

924. Coscia, L., et al. General pharmacological properties of p-phenetidine-α-N-n-propylpropionamide (FC 379). Arch. int. Pharmacodyn. 164:340-344, 1966.

925. Essman, W. B. Anticonvulsive properties of xylocaine in mice susceptible to audiogenic seizures. Arch. int. Pharmacodyn. 164:376-386, 1966.

926. Mitchell, C. L. The effect of drugs on the latency for an escape response elicited by electrical stimulation of the tooth pulp in cats. Arch. int. Pharmacodyn. 164:427-433, 1966.

927. Hill, H. E., et al. Comparative effects of methadone, meperidine and morphine on conditioned suppression. Arch. int. Pharmacodyn. 163:341-352, 1966.

928. Marazzi-Uberti, E. and C. Turba. α-isopropyl-α-(2-dimethylaminoethyl)-1-naphylacetamide (naphthpyramide, DA 992): a new anti-inflammatory agent. I. Anti-inflammatory activity and acute toxicity. Arch. int. Pharmacodyn. 162:378-397, 1966.

929. Hanson, H. M., et al. Estimation of relative antiavoidance activity of depressant drugs in squirrel monkeys. Arch. int. Pharmacodyn. 161:7-16, 1966.

930. Dashputra, P. G., et al. Modification of metrazol induced convulsions in rats by antihistaminics. Arch. int. Pharmacodyn. 160: 106-112, 1966.

931. Weiss, B. and V. G. Laties. Changes in pain tolerance and other behavior produced by salicylates. J. Pharmacol. Exp. Therap. 131:120-129, 1961.

932. Aceto, M. D., et al. Effects of drugs on conditioning in the rat. J. Pharm. Sci. 56: 823-827, 1961.

933. Kuhn, W. L. and E. F. Van Maanen. Central nervous system affects of thalidomide. J. Pharmacol. Exp. Therap. 134:60-68, 1961.

934. Kelleher, R. T., et al. Effects of meprobamate on operant behavior in rats. J. Pharmacol. Exp. Therap. 133:271-280, 1961.

935. Bastian, J. W. Classification of CNS drugs by a mouse screening battery. Arch. int. Pharmacodyn. 133:347-364, 1961.

936. Becker, B. A. Pharmacologic activity of phentermine (phenyl-t-butylamine). Toxicol. Appl. Pharmacol. 3:256-259, 1961.

937. Cho, M. H. Quantitation of spontaneous movements of animals given psychotropic drugs. J. Appl. Physiol. 16:390-391, 1961.

938. Dresse, A. and C. Niemengeers. Is the stimulation of certain nervous centers by apomorphine subject to tachyphylaxis? Comt. Rend. Soc. Biol. 155:1713-1715, 1961.

939. Fischer, E. and M. Lopez Amalfara. Effects of catechol amines on the motor behavior of lauchas (rodents) and their modification by adrenergic blocking. Ciencia Invest. (Buenos Aires) 17:138-140, 1961.

940. Kameyama, T. Studies on analgesics. VI. Analgesic activity of sympathomimetic amines and other drugs. Yakugaku Zasshi 81:215-221, 1961.

941. Linyuchev, M. N., et al. Restoration with phenamine (amphetamine) of conditioned reflexes deranged through the use of cholinolytics. Farmakol. i Toksikol. 24:659-664, 1961.

942. Mantegazza, P. and M. Riva. Anorexigenic activity of L (-) DOPA in animals pretreated with monoaminoxidase inhibitor. Med. Exptl. 4:367-373, 1961.

943. Petkov, W. The mechanism of action of Panax ginseng C. A. Mey. The problem of the pharmacology of response mechanisms. Arzneimittel-Forsch. 11:288-295, 1961.

944. van Andel, H. and A. M. Ernst. Tryptamine-catatonia, a cholinergic hypofunction in the central nervous system. Psychopharmacologia 2:461-466, 1961.

945. White, R. P., et al. Phylogenetic comparison of central actions produced by different doses of atropine and hyoscine. Arch. int. Pharmacodyn. 132:349-363, 1961.

946. Fujimura, H., et al. Pharmacological action of 2-anilinoacetamide derivatives. Yakugaku Zasshi 81:659-663, 1961.

947. Vorobiova, T. M. Effect of small doses of various pharmacological preparations on conditioned reflexes in dogs. Fiziol. Zh. Akad. Nauk Ukr. RSR 7:24-31, 1961.

948. Silvestrini, B. and C. Pozzatti. Pharmacological properties of 3-phenyl-5-diethylaminoethyl-1,2,4-oxadiazole. Brit. J. Pharmacol. 16:209-217, 1961.

949. Vernier, V. G. The pharmacology of antidepressant agents. Diseases Nervous System 22:7-13, 1961.

950. Sabelli, H. C., et al. Cholinergic mechanisms and antidepressive agents. Rev. Soc. Arg. Biol. 37:87-92, 1961.

951. Kudrin, A. N. and L. P. Kokina. Effect of somniferous agents and of their combination with pentamin on the external inhibition of positive conditioned food reflexes. Farmikol. i Toksikol. 24:397-403, 1961.

952. Steinberg, H., et al. Modification of the effects of an amphetamine-barbiturate mixture by the past experience of rats. Nature 192:533-535, 1961.

953. Muller-Calgan, H. and R. Hotovy. Behavioral changes in the cat in response to various drugs acting as stimulants of the central nervous system. Arzneimittel-Forsch. 11:642-649, 1961.

954. Vane, J. R., et al. Tryptamine receptors in the central nervous system. Nature 191:1068-1069, 1961.

955. Chen, G. and B. Bohner. Anticonvulsant properties of 1-(1-phenylcyclohexyl) piperidine-HCl and certain other drugs. Proc. Soc. Exptl. Biol Med. 106:632-635, 1961.

956. Child, K. J., et al. Some effects of reserpine on barbitone anesthesia in mice. Biochem. Pharmacol. 6:252-256, 1961.

957. Fukushima, K. Experimental studies on the drugs of antishock. Kagoshima Daigaku Igaku Zasshi. 13:416-437, 1961.

958. Kita, T., et al. Studies on central depressants. I. Pharmacological activity of γ-substituted butyric acid derivatives. Yakugaku Kenkyu 33:36-47, 1961.

959. Bentley, G. A. The susceptibility of rats to audiogenic seizures following acute and prolonged medication with narcotic drugs. Arch. int. Pharmacodyn. 132:378-391, 1961.

960. Greenblatt, E. N. and A. C. Osterberg. Correlations of activating and lethal effects of excitatory drugs in grouped and isolated mice. J. Pharmacol. Exp. Therap. 131:115-119, 1961.

961. Shuster, V., et al, Pharmacological data on the analeptic benegrade. Latvijas PSR Zinatm Akad. Vestis, No. 8:105-110, 1961.

962. Maffii, G., et al. A new analeptic: 5,5-diethyl-1,3-oxazin-2,4-dione (dioxone). J. Pharmacol. 13:244-253, 1961.

963. Nicholls, P. J. Pharmacological properties of some β-glutarimides. Arch. int. Pharmacodyn. 133:212-235, 1961.

964. Zbinden, G., et al. Experimental and clinical toxicology of chlorodiazepoxide (Librium). Toxicol. Appl. Pharmacol. 3:619-637, 1961.

965. Kuriyama, K. Electroencephalographic studies on the antagonism between β,β-methylethylglutarimide and some kinds of anesthetics. Nippon Yakurigaku Zasshi 57:560-565, 1961.

966. Hahn, F., et al. The effect of bemegrid, noradrenalin and artificial respiration on thiopental anesthesia in dogs. Arch. Exptl. Pathol. Pharakol. 242:168-187, 1961.

967. Denisenko, P. P. The effect of cholinolytics, chiefly acting on the central nervous system, on conditioned reflex activity in rabbits. Pavlov J. Higher Nervous Activity 11:113-118, 1961.

968. Ilyuchenok, R. Y. and M. D. Mashkovskii. Correlation of anticholinesterase substances (galanthamine and eserine) with choline-and adreno-lytics in the region of the reticular formation in the brain stem. Farmakol. i Toksikol. 24:403-410, 1961.

969. Denisenko, P. P. The antagonistic action of cholinomimetic and central cholinolytic agents on the EEG of the rabbit. Seckenov Physiol. J. USSR 47:124-131, 1961.

970. Sergio, C. The effect of bulbocapnine on EEG and flight reaction by hypothalmic stimulation in rabbits. Riv. Neurobiol. 7: 451-462, 1961.

971. Van Harreveld, A. and J. E. Bogen. The clinging position of the bulbocapninized cat. Exptl. Neurol. 4:241-261, 1961.

972. Hughes, F. W. and R. B. Forney. Alcohol and caffeine in choice-discrimination tests in rats. Proc. Soc. Exptl. Biol. Med. 108: 157-159, 1961.

973. Sommer, S. and R. Hotovy. Differentiation of the central stimulating action of 2-ethyl-amino-3-phenyl-norcomphane. Arznemittel-Forsch. 11:969-972, 1961.

974. Gerber, C. J. Effect of selected excitant and depressant agents on the cortical response to midline thalamic stimulation in the rabbit. Electroencephalog. Clin. Neurophysiol. 13:354-364, 1961.

975. Carroll, M. N., Jr., et al. The pharmacology of a new oxazolidimon with anticonvulsant, analgetic and muscle relaxant properties. Arch. Inter. Pharmacodyn. 130: 280-298, 1961.

976. Baruk, H. and J. Launay. Experimental psychotropic action of chlorodiazepoxide in the monkey. Practical consequences in human therapy. Ann. Medicopsychol. 119: 957-962, 1961.

977. Randall, L. O., et al. Pharmacological and clinical studies on Valium, a new psychotherapeutic agent of the benzodiazepine class. Current Therap. Res. 3:405-425, 1961.

978. Frommel, E., et al. What is the place of morphine and cocaine in the armamentarium of the so-called psychopharmacological drugs? Schweiz. Med. Wochschr. 91:1102-1108, 1961.

979. Nikitina, G. M. The effect of chlorpromazine on the interrelation of motor and autonomic components of the conditioned defense reaction in animals during ontogenesis. Pavlov J. Higher Nervous Activity 11:98-104, 1961.

980. Khrabrova, O. P. Specific features of the animal reaction to a shock-inducing stimulus following the administration of aminazine. Bull. Exptl. Biol. Med. 51:147-150, 1961.

981. Smith, M. E., et al. Psychotherapeutic agents and ethyl alcohol. Quart. J. Studies Alc. 22:241-249, 1961.

982. Faenzi, C. Effect of neuraleptic and relaxant drugs in convulsive states induced by toxic doses of local anesthetics. Boll. Soc. Ital. Biol. Sper. 39:414-417, 1961.

983. Lambert, P. A., et al. Notes on the neuroleptic inactivity of a phenothiazine derivative with pure antiapomorphine properties. Pharmacodynamic and clinical study of 3-dimethyl-sulfamoyl-10-[3-(1-methylsulfonyl-4-piperazino)-propyl] phenothiazine (R.P. 9,260). Psychopharmacologia 2:209-213, 1961.

984. Schuette, D. V. and W. L. Gulick. The effects of chlorpromazine upon the ear and the VIII cranial nerve. Ann. Otol. Rhinol. Laryngol. 70:143-163, 1961.

985. Wu, Hsi-Jui. The action mechanism of reserpine compared with that of certain other tranquilizing substances. Bull. Exptl. Biol. Med. 51:461-465, 1961.

986. Bienfet, V., et al. Pharmacologic assay of dixyrazine. Acta Neurol. Psychiat. Belg. 61: 669-685, 1961.

987. Knoll, J. Motimeter, a new sensitive apparatus for the quantitative measurement of hypermotility caused by psychostimulants. Arch. int. Pharmacodyn. 130:141-154, 1961.

988. Maxwell, D. R. and H. T. Palmer. Demonstration of anti-depressant or stimulant properties of imipramine in experimental animals. Nature 191:84-85, 1961.

989. Cahen, R. The pharmacology of pholcodine. Bull. Narcotics U.N. Dept. Social Affairs 13: 19-36, 1961.

990. Pinto Corrado, A. and V. G. Longo. An electrophysiological analysis of the convulsant action of morphine, codeine and thebaine. Arch. int. Pharmacodyn. 132:255-269, 1961.

991. Frommell, E., et al. The pharmacodynamics of the anilide of (pyrrolidino-N)-3-N-butyric acids (WS 10), a basal neuroleptic and cortical thymoleptic drug. Arch. int. Pharmacodyn. 130:235-259, 1961.

992. Harris, L. S. and F. C. Uhle. Enhancement of amphetamine stimulation and prolongation of barbiturate depression by a substituted pyrid [3,4-6] indole derivative. J. Pharmacol. Exp. Therap. 132:251-257, 1961.

993. Crampton, G. H. Habituation of vestibular nystagmus in the cat during sustained arousal produced by d-amphetamine. U.S. Army Medical Research Lab. Ft. Knox, Kentucky, Rept. No. 488, Aug. 18, 1961.

994. McLennan, H. The effect of some catecholamines upon a monosynaptic reflex pathway in the spinal cord. J. Physiol. 158:411-425, 1961.

995. Goldstein, L. and C. Muñoz. Influence of adrenergic stimulant and blocking drugs on cerebral electrical activity in curarized animals. J. Pharmacol. Exp. Therap. 132: 345-353, 1961.

996. Takahashi, R., et al. Relationship of ammonia and acetylcholine levels to brain excitability. J. Neurochem. 7:103-112, 1961.

997. Bastian, J. W. and G. R. Clements. Pharmacology and toxicology of hydroxyphenamate (Listica). Diseases Nervous System Suppl. 22:9-16, 1961.

998. Van Tai-An and M. G. Belekhova. The influences of the cervical sympathetic nerve and the effects of some pharmacological substances on the "recruitment reaction." Secherov. Physiol J. USSR 47:18-29, 1961.

999. Kita, T. and H. Kamiya. Central depressant. II. Several methods of screening γ-aminobutyric acid derivatives by mouse behavior. Yakugaku Kenkyu 33:758-766, 1961.

1000. Busche, E. Test of spinal reflexes and neuromuscular transmission in decerebrate rats and of the effect of muscle relaxants on them. Arch. int. Pharmacodyn. 132:139-146, 1961.

1001. Vacek, L. A study on steroid anesthesia: 6. The effect of serotonin and its antagonists on the central inhibiting effect of hydroxypreguanedione. Scripta Med. Fac. Med. Univ. Brun. Olomuc. 34:65-72, 1961.

1002. Levis, S., et al. Pharmacological characteristics of a new tranquilizing agent: Dixyrazine. Arch. int. Pharmacodyn. 131:262-282, 1961.

1003. Herr, F., et al. Tranquilizers and antidepressants: a pharmacological comparison. Arch. int. Pharmacodyn. 134:328-342, 1961.

1004. Rubio-Chevamier, H., et al. Potentiating action of imipramine upon "reticular arousal." Exptl. Neurol. 4:214-220, 1961.

1005. Crepax, P., et al. Effects of imipramine on cerebral electrical phenomena in the cat due to activation of thalamo-cortical, transcallosal and intracortical circuits. Boll. Soc. Ital. Biol. Sper. 37:180-183, 1961.

1006. Himwich, W. A. and J. C. Petersen. Effect of the combined administration of imipramine and a monoamine oxidase inhibitor. Am. J. Psychiat. 117:928-929, 1961.

1007. Muller-Calgan, H. and R. Hotovy. Behavioral changes in the cat in response to various drugs acting as stimulants of the central nervous system. Arzneimittel-Forsch. 11:642-649, 1961.

1008. Pfeifer, A. F., et al. Effect of tranquilizing drugs on the pharmacological actions of diethyltryptamine. Acta physiol. Acad. Sci. Hung. 19:225-233, 1961.

1009. Schallek, W., et al. Effects of chlordiazepoxide (Librium) and other psychotropic agents on the limbic system of the brain. Ann. N. Y. Acad. Sci. 96:303-312, 1961.

1010. Acheson, R. M., et al. Attempted correlations between behavioral and biochemical changes in rats following reserpine and chronic administration of amine-oxidase inhibitors. Psychopharmacologia 2:277-294, 1961.

1011. Angelucci, L. Analgesia without respiratory depression by means of association of morphine, structural antagonists and Daptazol. Minerva Anestesiologia 27:216-222, 1961.

1012. Berry, C. A., et al. A comparison of the anticonvulsant activity of mepivacain and lidocain. J. Pharmacol. Exp. Therap. 133: 357-363, 1961.

1013. Dhawan, B. N. and G. P. Gupta. Antiemetic activity of D-lysergic acid diethylamide. J. Pharmacol. Exp. Therap. 133: 137-139, 1961.

1014. Fluckiger, E. and R. Salzmann. Serotonin antagonism (observed) on the placenta. Experientia 17:131, 1961.

1015. Ueki, S., et al. Effects of mecamylamine on the Golgi recurrent collateral-Renshaw-cell synapse in the spinal cord. Exptl. Neurol. 3:141-148, 1961.

1016. Burke, J. C. The muscle relaxant properties of 2,2-dichloro-1-(p-chlorophenyl)-1,3-propanediol-O^3-carbamate. Arch. int. Pharmacodyn. 134:216-223, 1961

1017. Gross, C. G. and L. Weiskrantz. The effect of the "tranquilizers" on auditory discrimination and delayed response performance of monkeys. Quart. J. Exptl. Psychol 13:34-39, 1961.

1018. Gray, W. D., et al. Neuropharmacological actions of mephenoxalone. Arch. int. Pharmacodyn. 134:198-215, 1961.

1019. Frommel, E., et al. Meprobamate, phenobarbitol, or meprobamate plus phenobarbital. Anais Azevedos (Lisbon) 13:184-207, 1961.

1020. Inoki, R., et al. Comparison of the action of related compounds of Soma. Nippon Yakurigaku Zaschi 57:280-288, 1961.

1021. Jacob, J. and M. Blozovski. Effects of various analgesic agents on the behavior of mice subjected to a thermoalgesic stimulus. II. Learning under nociceptive stress conditions. Comparative effects of analgesic and psychoactive agents on licking and leaping reactions. Arch. int. Pharmacodyn. 133:296-309, 1961.

1022. Maxwell, D. R., et al. A comparison of the analgesic and some other central properties of methotromeprazine and morphine. Arch. int. Pharmacodyn. 132:60-73, 1961.

1023. Kikutomo, T. The electroencephalogram of rabbits under the influence of reserpine and the effects of methamphetamine. Nippon Yakurigaku Zasshi 57:173-192, 1961.

1024. Faidherbe, J., et al. Differential action of a central nervous stimulant demonstrated by a technique of "operant" conditioning in the cat. Arch. Int. Physiol. Biochim. 69: 52-68, 1961.

1025. Szporny, L. and P. Gorog. Investigations into the correlations between monoamine oxidase inhibition and other effects due to methylphenidate and its stereoisomers. Biochem. Pharmacol. 8:263-268, 1961.

1026. Farner, D. Studies on the effect of drugs on animals of various ages. IV. The effect of Ritalin and Regitin on young and old rats. Gerontologia 5:45-54, 1961.

1027. Shemano, I., et al. A pharmacological comparison of phenazocaine hydrobromide and morphine sulfate as narcotic analgesics. J. Pharmacol. Exp. Therap. 132:258-263, 1961.

1028. Martin, W. R. and C. G. Eades. Demonstration of tolerance and physical dependence in the dog following a short-term infusion of morphine. J. Pharmacol. Exp. Therap. 133: 262-270, 1961.

1029. Ohnesorge, F. K. and A. L. Khan. Effects of phenmetrozine on oxygen consumption and spontaneous motor activity. Arzneimittel-Forsch. 11:793-795, 1961.

1030. Janssen, P. A. J. Pirinitramide (R3365), a potent analgesic with unusual chemical structure. J. Pharm. Pharmacol. 13:513-530, 1961.

1031. Hotovy, R., et al. Pharmacologic properties of 2-ethyl-amino-3-phenyl-norcamphane. Arznemittel-Forsch 11:20-29, 1967.

1032. Szegi, J., et al. New contributions to the antagonism of morphine and N-allynormorphine derivatives. Acta Physiol. Acad. Sci. Hung. 19:273-285, 1961.

1033. Witkin, L. B., et al. Pharmacology of 2-amino-indane hydrochloride (Su-8629): a potent non-narcotic analgesic. J. Pharmacol. Exp. Therap. 133:400-408, 1961.

1034. Mashkovskii, M. D. and R. Y. Ilyuchenok. The effect of galanthamine on the central nervous system. Zh. Nevropatol. i Pskhiatr. 61:166-175, 1961.

1035. P'an, S. Y., et al. Anticonvulsant effect of nialamide and diphenyl-hydantoin. Proc. Soc. Exptl. Biol. Med. 108:680-683, 1961.

1036. Cortes, J. L. and G. V. Villagran. Nialamide and anaphylactic and histamine shock in guinea pigs. Medicine 41:146-163, 1961.

1037. Lebeden, V. P. Effect of nicotine on proprioceptive reflexes. Farmakol. i Toksikol. 24:515-518, 1961.

1038. DaVanzo, J. P., et al. Anticonvulsant properties of amino-oxyacetic acid. Am. J. Physiol. 201:833-837, 1961.

1039. Ohashi, H. The relation between corticospinal electrical activity and convulsions produced by the intravenous injection of ammonium salts. Seishin Shinkeigaku Zasshi 63: 31-43, 1961.

1040. Janssen, P. A. J. Comparative pharmacological data on 6 new basic 4'-fluorobutyrophenone derivatives: haloperidol, haloanisone, triperidol, methylperidide, haloperidide, and dipiperone. Arzneimittel-Forsch 11:819-824, 1961.

1041. Tislow, R. Pharmacology and toxicity of carphenazine. Diseases Nervous System 22: 7-13, 1961.

1042. Alema, G., et al. Experimental catatonia induced by neuroleptic drugs. I. Action of phenothiazine derivatives. Boll. Soc. Ital. Biol. Sper. 37:1037-1040, 1961.

1043. O'Dell, T. B. Experimental parameters in the evaluation of analgesics. Chicago Med. 63: 9-15, 1961.

1044. Schneider, C. Effects of morphine-like drugs in chicks. Nature 191:607-608, 1961.

1045. Nilsen, P. L. Studies on algesimetry by electrical stimulation of the mouse tail. Acta Pharmacol. Toxicol. 18:10-22, 1961.

1046. Bovet-Nitti, F., et al. A new MAO inhibitor: N'-(1,4-benzodioxane-2-methyl)-N'-benzyl-hydrazine (2596 IS). Compt. Rend. 252:614-616, 1961.

1047. Frommel, E., et al. Pharmacodynamics of a new tranquilizer with relaxant and antitremor effects and prolonged action: Go 560, or 3-(γ-butoxy, β-carbamyl, β-propanol)-5-phenyl, 5-ethylmalonylurea. Experimental study. Helv. Physiol. Pharmacol. Acta 19: 241-253, 1961.

1048. Aston, R. and E. F. Domino. Differential effects of phenobarbital, pentobarbital, and diphenylhydantoin on motor cortical and reticular thresholds in the Rhesus monkey. Psychopharmacologia 2:304-317, 1961.

1049. Popova, E. N. Some data on eserine's effect on the cerebral cortex of white rats. Communication 1. The effect of eserine on conditioned reflex activity. Bull. Exptl. Biol. 51:198-203, 1961.

1050. Venulet, J. Correlation between antiserotonin and depressor action of some phenothiazine derivatives. Acta Physiol. Polan. 12: 281-290, 1961.

1051. Kucherenko, T. M. Changes in higher nervous activity in dogs under the influence of pirhydrol. Pavlov J. Higher Nervous Activity 11:64-69, 1961.

1052. Beaulness, A. and G. Viens. Catatonia and catalepsy. Rev. Can. Biol. 20:215-220, 1961.

1053. Geller, I. Behavioral procedures used in evaluation of the psychopharmacological effects of carphenazine. Diseases Nervous System Suppl. 22:19-22, 1961.

1054. Logerspetz, K. and R. Tirri. The induction of physiological tolerance to promazine in mice. Ann. Med. Exptl. Biol. Fenniae Suppl. 5, 39:1-24, 1961.

1055. Decsi, L. Further studies on the metabolic background of tranquilizing drug action. Psychopharmacologia 2:224-242, 1961.

1056. Tedeschi, D. H., et al. Interaction of neuroleptics with serotonin in the central nervous system. Rev. Can. Biol. 20:209-214, 1961.

1057. Ilyuchenok, R. Y. and R. U. Ostrovskaia. The effect of diprazine on the bioelectric activity of the brain. Formakol. i Toksikol. 24:18-22, 1961.

1058. Laborit, H., et al. An experimental "excitation-hypotonic" syndrome. Arch. int. Pharmacodyn. 131:151-163, 1961.

1059. Menge, H. G. Experimental studies with animals on the central stimulating effect of a new theophilline derivative. Arzneimittel-Forsch. 11:271-273, 1961.

1060. Melson, F. Pharmacological study of some derivatives of 1,3-dioxolane with special reference to their actions on the central nervous system. Acta Biol. Med. Ger. 6:395-406, 1961.

1061. Herz, A. Influence of anticholinergic, nicotinolytic and antihistaminic drugs on the central inhibitory and stimulating morphine effects in the rat. Arch. Exptl. Pathol. Pharmakol. 241:236-253, 1961.

1062. Knoll, J., et al. Experimental analysis of the central effect of convulsive hydrazines. Acta Physiol. Acad. Sci. Hung. 19:169-178, 1961.

1063. Voss, E., et al. Reduction of tetramine toxicity by sedatives and anti-convulsants. J. Pharm. Sci. 50:858-860, 1961.

1064. Melander, B. and G. Gliniecke. Amphetamine, diethylpropion and tronylcypromin, a psychopharmacological study in the relation between structure and activity. Acta Pharmacol. Toxicol. 18:239-248, 1961.

1065. Costa, E. and G. R. Pscheidt. Correlations between active eyelid closure and depletion of brain biogenic amines by reserpine. Proc. Soc. Exptl. Biol. Med. 106:693-696, 1961.

1066. Decsi, L., et al. Tolerance to tremorine. Acta Physiol. Acad. Sci. Hung. 18:353-356, 1961.

1067. Arrigo, A., et al. Electroencephalographic study of the central action of yohimbine and yohimbic acid. Boll. Soc. Ital. Biol. Sper. 37:787-790, 1961.

1068. Baxter, B. L. The effect of selected drugs on the "emotional" behavior elicited via hypothalamic stimulation. Int. J. Neuropharmacol. 7:47-54, 1968.

1069. Olds, M. E. and G. Baldrighi. Effects of meprobamate, chlorodiazepoxide, diazepam, and sodium pentobarbital on visually evoked responses in the tectotegmental area of the rat. Int. J. Neuropharmacol. 7:231-239, 1968.

1070. Miyasaka, M. and E. F. Domino. Neuronal mechanisms of ketamine-induced anesthesia. Int. J. Neuropharmacol. 7:557-573, 1968.

1071. Barnett, A., et al. Activity of antihistamines in laboratory antidepressant tests. Int. J. Neuropharmacol. 8:73-79, 1969.

1072. Christmas, A. J. and D. R. Maxwell. A comparison of the effects of some benzodiazepines and other drugs on aggressive and exploratory behavior in mice and rats. Neuropharmacol. 9:17-29, 1970.

1073. Chen, G., et al. The neuropharmacology of 2-(o-chlorophenyl)-2-methylaminocyclohexanone hydrochloride. J. Pharmaco. Exp. Therap. 152:332-339, 1966.

1074. Tobia, A. J., et al. Altered reflex vasodilatation in the hypertensive rat: Possible role of histamine. J. Pharmacol. Exp. Therap. 175:619-626, 1970.

1075. Downes, H., et al. A study of the excitatory effects of barbiturates. J. Pharmacol. Exp. Therap. 175:692-699, 1970.

1076. Büch, H., et al. Stereospecificity of anesthetic activity, distribution, inactivation, and protein binding of the optical antipodes of two N-methylated barbiturates. J. Pharmacol. Exp. Therap. 175:703-716, 1970.

1077. Nigrovic, V., et al. Diuretic response to mercuric cysteine: Dependency on urinary pH. J. Pharmacol. Exp. Therap. 175:741-748, 1970.

1078. Dren, A. T. and E. F. Domino. Effects of hemicholinium (HC-3) on EEG activation and brain acetylcholine in the dog. J. Pharmacol. Exp. Therap. 161:141-154, 1968.

1079. Levin, J. A., et al. Active reflex vasodilatation induced by intravenous epinephrine or norepinephrine in primates. J. Pharmacol. Exp. Therap. 161:262-270, 1968.

1080. Pfeiffer, C. C., et al. Comparative study of the effect of meprobamate on the conditioned response on strychnine and pentylenetetrazol thresholds, on the normal electroencephalogram and on polysynaptic reflexes. Ann. N.Y. Acad. Sci. 67:734-745, 1957.

1081. Lish, P. M., et al. Mode of the bronchodilator action of Phentolamine. J. Pharmacol. Exp. Therap. 163:11-16, 1968.

1082. Brown, J. H., et al. Oral effectiveness of beta adrenergic antagonists in preventing epinephrine-induced metabolic responses. J. Pharmacol. Exp. Therap. 163:25-35, 1968.

1083. Kvam, D. C., et al. Effect of some new β-adrenergic blocking agents on certain metabolic responses to catecholamines. J. Pharmacol. Exp. Therap. 149:183-192, 1965.

1084. Dungan, K. W., et al. Pharmacologic potency and selectivity of a new bronchodilator agent: Soterenol (MJ 1992). J. Pharmacol. Exp. Therap. 164:290-301, 1968.

1085. Miranda, P. M. S., et al. Vasodilatation of brainstem origin suppressed by neuromuscular blockade in the cat. J. Pharmacol. Exp. Therap. 164:333-341, 1968.

1086. Weinstock, M. and A. S. Marshall. The influence of the sympathetic nervous system on the action of drugs on the lens. J. Pharmacol. Exp. Therap. 166:8-13, 1969.

1087. Friedman, M. J. and J. H. Jaffee. A central hypothermic response to pilocarpine in the mouse. J. Pharmacol. Exp. Therap. 167: 34-44, 1969.

1088. McKenna, D. H., et al. Effect of propranolol on systemic and coronary hemodynamics at rest and during simulated exercise. Circ. Res. 19:520-527, 1966.

1089. Lucchesi, B. R. The effects of pronethalol and its dextro isomer upon experimental cardiac arrhythmias. J. Pharmacol. Exp. Therap. 148:94-99, 1965.

1090. Parmley, W. W. and E. Braunwald. Comparative myocardial depressant and antiarrhythmic properties of d-propranol, dl-propranolol and quinidine. J. Pharmacol. Exp. Therap. 158:11-21, 1967.

1091. Giudicelli, J.-F., et al. Studies on dl-4-(2-hydroxy-3-isopropylaminopropoxy)-indole (LB 46), a new potent β-adrenergic blocking drug. J. Pharmacol. Exp. Therap. 168:116-126, 1969.

1092. Stitzer, M., et al. Effects of nicotine on fixed interval behavior and their modification by cholinergic antagonists. J. Pharmacol. Exp. Therap. 171:166-177, 1970.

1093. Carlson, G. M., et al. Effects of nicotine on gastric antral and duodenal contractile activity in the dog. J. Pharmacol. Exp. Therap. 172:367-376, 1970.

1094. Alexander, G. J., et al. Lysergic acid diethylamide intake in pregnancy: Fetal damage in rats. J. Pharmacol. Exp. Therap. 173:48-59, 1970.

1095. Kubena, R. K. and H. Barry, III. Interactions of Δ'-tetrahydrocannibinol with barbiturates and methamphetamine. J. Pharmacol. Exp. Therap. 173:94-100, 1970.

1096. Killam, K. F., et al. An animal model of light sensitive epilepsy. Electroencephalogr. Clin. Neurophysiol. 22:497-513, 1967.

1097. Stark, L. G., et al. The anticonvulsant effects of phenobarbital, diphenylhydantoin and two benzodiazepines in the baboon. Papio papio. J. Pharmacol. Exp. Therap. 173:125-132, 1970.

1098. Baker, R. G. and E. G. Anderson. The effects of L-3,4-dihydroxyphenylalanine on spinal reflex activity. J. Pharmacol. Exp. Therap. 173:212-223, 1970.

1099. Herz, A., et al. Central nicotine- and muscarinelike properties of cholinomimetic drugs with regard to their lipid solubilities. Ann. N. Y. Acad. Sci. 142:21-26, 1967.

1100. Vazquez, A. J. and J. E. P. Toman. Some interactions of nicotine with other drugs upon central nervous function. Ann. N. Y. Acad. Sci. 142:201-215, 1967.

1101. Morrison, C. F. and A. K. Armitage. Effects of nicotine upon the free operant behavior of rats and spontaneous motor activity of mice. Ann. N. Y. Acad. Sci. 142: 268-276, 1967.

1102. Kadzielawa, K. and E. Widy. The influence of imipramine on the central effects of dihydroxyphenylalanine. Neuropharmacol. 9: 467-480, 1970.

1103. Banna, N. R. and S. J. Jabbur. The action of bemegrade on presynaptic inhibition. Neuropharmacol. 9:553-560, 1970.

1104. Kirkpatrick, W. E. and P. Lomax. Temperature changes induced by chlorpromazine and n-methyl chlorpromazine in the rat. Neuropharmacol. 10:61-66, 1971.

1105. Fuentes, J. A. and V. G. Longo. An investigation on the central effects of harmine, harmaline and related β-carbolines. Neuropharmacol. 10:15-23, 1971.

1106. Peterson, A. E. and C. N. Gillis. Pharmacological alteration of cardiovascular changes secondary to hypothalamic stimulation in rats. Fed. Proc. 29:741, 1970.

1107. Korol, B. and M. L. Brown. A behavioral and autonomic nervous system study of RO-5-3350 and diazepam in conscious dogs. Pharmacol. 1:115-128, 1968.

1108. Yen, H. C. Y., et al. Effects of some psychoactive drugs on experimental 'neurotic' (conflict induced) behavior in cats. Pharmacol 3:32-40, 1970.

1109. Evangelista, A. M., et al. Effect of amphetamine, nicotine, and hexamethonium on performance of a conditioned response during acquisition and retention trials. Pharmacol. 3:91-96, 1970.

1110. Schueler, F. W. The mechanism of action of the hemicholiniums. Int. Rev. Neurobiol. 2:77-97, 1960.

1111. Lomax, P. Drugs and body temperature. Int. Rev. Neurobiol. 12:1-43, 1970.

1112. Singh, K. P. and M. M. Mahawar. Some inhibitory actions of catecholamines and their blockade by propranolol. Arch. Int. Pharmacodyn. 171:58-67, 1968.

1113. Mazurkiewicz, I. M. The effects of β-adrenergic receptor blockade on the blood pressure and heart rate changes induced by noradrenaline infusion and postinfusional hypotension. Arch. int. Pharmacodyn. 171: 136-158, 1968.

1114. Rodriguez, R. and E. G. Pardo. Drug reversal of pain induced functional impairment. Arch. int. Pharmacodyn. 172:148-160, 1968.

1115. Chen, G., et al. Studies of drug effects on electrically induced extensor seizures and clinical implications. Arch. int. Pharmacodyn. 172:183-218, 1968.

1116. Cohen, M. and H. Wakeley. A comparative behavioral study of ditran and LSD in mice, rats, and dogs. Arch. int. Pharmacodyn. 173: 316-326, 1968.

1117. Straw, R. N. The effect of certain benzodiazepines on the threshold for pentylenetetrazol-induced seizures in the cat. Arch. int. Pharmacodyn. 175:464-469, 1968.

1118. Dandiya, P. C. and L. P. Bhargava. The antiparkinsonian activity of monoamine oxidase inhibitors and other agents in rats and mice. Arch. int. Pharmacodyn. 176:157-167, 1968.

1119. Weller, C. P., et al. Analgesic profile of tranquilizers in multiple screening tests in mice. Arch. int. Pharmacodyn. 177:287-289, 1968.

1120. Erill, S. Persistence of the hypoglycemic effect of tolbutamide after block of β-adrenergic receptors. Arch. int. Pharmacodyn. 177: 88-91, 1969.

1121. Ganesan, D. Influence of female sex hormones on pentobarbitone sodium anesthesia in rats. Arch. int. Pharmacodyn. 177:88-91, 1969.

1122. Bernauer, W., et al. Comparison of the antilethal, broncholytic, and antiemphysematous activities of mepyramine in anaphylactic, histamine, and anaphylatoxin shock of guinea pigs. Arch. int. Pharmacodyn. 178:137-151, 1969.

1123. Randall, L. O., et al. Pharmacological studies on fluazepam hydrochloride (RO5-6901), a new psychotropic agent of the benzodiazepine class. Arch. int. Pharmacodyn. 178: 216-241, 1969.

1124. Marchetti, E. Pharmacological activities of a new antitussive agent: Morphethylbutyne. Arch. int. Pharmacodyn. 178:400-406, 1969.

1125. Wardell, J. R., Jr., and R. G. Staples, III. Animal studies comparing the neuropharmacological profile of a trifluoperazine HCl-amobarbital combination with that of the individual components. Arch. int. Pharmacodyn. 179: 106-120, 1969.

1126. McClure, D. A. 4-Dimethyl-amino methyl-2-methyl 1,3-dioxolane—a new potent analgesic agent. Arch. int. Pharmacodyn. 179:154-160, 1969.

1127. Yamamoto, J. and A. Sekiya. On the pressor action of propanolol in the rat. Arch. int. Pharmacodyn. 179:372-380, 1969.

1128. Stockhaus, K. und H. Wick. Toxizitätsunterschiede von pharmaka bei subcutaner, intragastraler und intraduodenaler applikation bei Ratten. Arch. int. Pharmacodyn. 180:155-161, 1969.

1129. Molinengo, L. and S. Ricci Gamalero. Behavioral action and tranquillizing effects of reserpine, diazepam and hydroxyzine. Arch. int. Pharmacodyn. 180:217-231, 1969.

1130. Chopra, Y. M. and P. C. Dandiya. On the mechanism of reversal of reserpine action by pargyline hydrochloride. Arch. int. Pharmacodyn. 181:47-56, 1969.

1131. Carminati, G. M. Attivita comparata di svariatifarmaci in alcuni tests sperimentali di studio del comportamento. Arch. int. Pharmacodyn. 181:68-93, 1969.

1132. Blum, K. The effect of dopamine and other catecholamines on neuromuscular transmission. Arch. int. Pharmacodyn. 181:297-306, 1969.

1133. Parra, J. and H. Vidrio. Drug effects on the blood pressure response to postural changes in the unanesthetized rabbit. Arch. int. Pharmacodyn. 181:353-362, 1969.

1134. Barrett, W. E., et al. Pharmacological investigation of a new orally active antiarrhythmic drug Su-13197. Arch. int. Pharmacodyn. 182:65-77, 1969.

1135. Isem, G. E., et al. A comparison of the lethal and respiratory effects of morphine in Long-Evans and Sprague-Dawley rats. Arch. int. Pharmacodyn. 182:130-138, 1969.

1136. Voith, K. and F. Herr. Psychopharmacological evaluation of a new antidepressant: butriptyline. Arch. int. Pharmacodyn. 182: 318-331, 1969.

1137. Pickering, R. W. A method for the quantitative assessment of compounds affecting respiration in conscious mice: effect of four selected respiratory stimulants. Arch. int. Pharmacodyn. 183:12-15, 1970.

1138. Salmon, G. K. and J. D. Ireson. A correlation between the hypotensive action of methyldopa and its depression of peripheral sympathetic function. Arch. int. Pharmacodyn. 183: 60-64, 1970.

1139. Rosenblum, W. I. Antihypertensive effect of nylidrin HCl. Arch. int. Pharmacodyn. 183: 85-92, 1970.

1140. Rosic, N. Partial antagonism by cholinesterase reactivators of the effects of organophosphate compounds on shuttle-box avoidance. Arch. int. Pharmacodyn. 183:139-147, 1970.

1141. Oliver, J. H., et al. Effect of reserpine and other drugs on the CNS and lethal effects of hyperbaric oxygen on mice. Arch. int. Pharmacodyn. 183:215-223, 1970.

1142. Chernov, H. I., et al. Pharmacological properties of Su-19789B, or unique central nervous system stimulant. Arch. int. Pharmacodyn. 184:34-44, 1970.

1143. Cloutier, G., et al. Evaluation pharmacodynamique d'un nouveau curarisant de synthese: la gallamine-acetylenique. Arch. int. Pharmacodyn. 184:75-92, 1970.

1144. Malick, J. B. and M. E. Goldberg. Effects of a choline acetyltransferase inhibitor on self-stimulatory behavior in the rat. Arch. int. Pharmacodyn. 184:254-256, 1970.

1145. Weinreich, D. and L. D. Clark. Anticonvulsant drugs and self-stimulation rates in rats. Arch. int. Pharmacodyn. 185:269-273, 1970.

1146. Lumachi, B., et al. Comparative pharmacological investigations on naphthypramide and some anti-inflammatory and skeletal muscle relaxant agents. Arch. int. Pharmacodyn. 186: 66-83, 1970.

1147. Malick, J. B. Effects of selected drugs on stimulus-bound emotional behavior elicited by hypothalamic stimulation in the cat. Arch. int. Pharmacodyn. 186:137-141, 1970.

1148. Hudson, R. D. and M. K. Wolpert. Anticonvulsant and motor depressant effects of diazepam. Arch. int. Pharmacodyn. 186:388-401, 1970.

1149. Feinstein, M. B., et al. The antagonism of local anesthetic induced convulsions by the benzodiazepine derivative diazepam. Arch. int. Pharmacodyn. 187:144-154, 1970.

1150. Longo, V. G., et al. Effects of nicotine on the electroencephalogram of the rabbit. Ann. N. Y. Acad. Sci. 142:159-169, 1967.

1151. Brown, B. B. Relationship between evoked response changes and behavior following small doses of nicotine. Ann. N. Y. Acad. Sci. 142: 190-200, 1967.

1152. Leszkovsky, G. and L. J. Tardos. Some effects of propranolol on the central nervous system. J. Pharm. Pharmacol. 17:518-519, 1965.

1153. Agarwal, S. L. and D. Bose. The role of brain catecholamines in drug induced tremor. Br. J. Pharmac. Chemother. 30:349-353, 1967.

1154. Korol, B. and M. L. Brown. The role of the β-adrenergic system in behavior: Antidepressant effects of propranolol. Curr. Therap. Res. 9:269-279, 197-.

1155. Aron, C., et al. Evaluation of a rapid technique for detecting minor tranquilizers. Neuropharmacol. 10:459-469, 1971.

1156. Nichols, R. E. and E. J. Walaszek. Antagonism of drug induced catatonia. Fed. Proc. 24: 390, 1965.

1157. Staff, Department of Pharmacology, University of Edinburgh. Pharmacological Experiments on Isolated Preparations E. and S. Livingstone Ltd. Edinburgh and London, 1968.

1158. Bohdanecky, Z., et al. The effect of neocortical and hippocampal spreading depression on the slow wave EEG activity induced by atropine. Arch. int. Pharmacodyn. 148:545-556, 1964.

1159. White, R. P., et al. Phylogenetic comparison of central actions produced by different doses of atropine and hyoscine. Arch. int. Pharmacodyn. 132:349-363, 1961.

1160. Wikler, A. Pharmacologic dissociation of behavior and EEG "Sleep Patterns" in dogs: Morphine, N-allylnormorphine and atropine. Proc. Soc. Exp. Biol. Med. 79:261-265, 1952.

1161. McGaugh, et al. Electroencephalographic and behavioral analysis of drug effects on an instrumental reward discrimination in rabbits. Psychopharmacologia 4:126-138, 1963.

1162. Rozhkova, E. K. Fiziologicheskaya rol atsetilkolinai izyskania novykh veshchesto in Mikhelson, M. Y. Len. Med. Inst. in Pavlova 230 pp 1957.

1163. Samuel, G. K., et al. Effects of scopolamine and atropine and their quaterniyed salts on avoidance behavior in monkey. Psychopharmacologia 8:205-301, 1965.

1164. Valenstein, E. S. A note on anesthetizing rats and Guinea pigs. J. Exp. Anal. Behav. 4: 6, 1961.

1165. Schallek, W. and A. Kuehn. Effects of benzodiazepines on spontaneous EEG and arousal responses of cats. Prog. in Brain Research 18:231-238, 1965.

1166. Rensch, B. and G. Ducker. Verzogerung de Vergessens erlernter visueller Aufgaben bei Tieren durch Chlorpromazin. Pflugers Archiv 289:200-214, 1966.

1167. Maickel, R., et al. Control of adipose tissue lipase activity by the sympathetic nervous system. Life. Sci. 3:210-214, 1963.

1168. Corson, S. A., et al. Ephedrine antagonism to behavioral and antidiuretic effects of reserpine. Fed. Proc. 24:197, 1965.

1169. Pscheidt, G. R., et al. Studies on norepinephrine and 5-hydroxytryptamine in various species. Comparative Neurochemistry. Charles Birchall and Sons, London, 1963.

1170. Pscheidt, G. R. and H. E. Himwich. Reserpine, monoamine oxidase inhibitors and distribution of biogenic amines in monkey brain. Biochem. Pharmacol. 12:65-71, 1963.

1171. Diamantis, W. and M. Kletzkin. Evaluation of muscle relaxant drugs by head-drop and by decerebrate rigidity. Int. J. Neuropharmicol. 5:305-310, 1966.

1172. Williams, B., et al. Electrical activity of the prepyriform cortex after reserpine in the rat. J. Pharmacol. Exp. Therap. 150:10-16, 1965.

1173. Meyers, B., et al. Some effects of muscarinic cholinergic blocking drugs on behavior and the electrocorticogram. Psychopharmacologia 5:289-300, 1964.

1174. Charney, N. H. and G. S. Reynolds. Development of behavioral compensation to the effects of scopolamine during fixed-interval reinforcement. J. Exptl. Anal. Behavior 8: 183-186, 1965.

1175. Motokizawa, F. and B. Fujimori. Arousal effect of afferent discharges from muscle spindles upon electroencephalograms in cats. Jap. J. Physiol. 14:344-353, 1964.

1176. Marsh, D. F. Pharmacological activity of 2-amino-5-chlorobenzoxazole (zoxazolamino, Flexin). II. Duration of action. Fed. Proc. 16: 319, 1957.

1177. Antonaccio, M. J. Reflex responses to vertical tilting in dogs: A comparison with bilateral carotid occulsion. Pharmacologist. 13:192, 1971.

1178. Winger, G. D., et al. Patterns of barbiturate-reinforced responding in the Rhesus monkey. Pharmacologist. 13:206, 1971.

1179. Cumming, J. F. Development of acute tolerance to Ketamine in the rat. Pharmacologist 13:212, 1971.

1180. Volicer, L. Effect of ethanol on adenosine 3',5'-monophosphate (cyclic AMP) in rat tissues invivo. Pharmacologist 13:213, 1971.

1181. Schleimer, R., et al. The anti-arrhythmic activity of dihydroergotamine (DHE). Pharmacologist 13:225, 1971.

1182. Hill, H. and A. Horita. Amphetamine-induced hyperthermia in rabbits. Pharmacologist 12:197, 1970.

1183. Tseng, L. F. and E. J. Walazek. Influence of alteration of catecholamine and serotonin levels on bulbocapnine-induced catatonia. Pharmacologist 12:198, 1970.

1184. Gessa, A., et al. Essential role of testosterone in the sexual stimulation induced by p-chlorophenylalanine (PCPA) in male animals. Pharmacologist 12:204, 1970.

1185. Hosko, M. J. and H. F. Hardman. Effect of Δ^9-THC on cardiovascular responses to stimulation of vasopressor loci in the neuraxis of anesthetized cats. Pharmacologist 13:296, 1971.

1186. Tagliamonte, P., et al. Differential effect of p-chlorophenylalanine (PCPA) on the sexual behavior and on the electrocorticogram of male rabbits. Pharmacologist 12:205, 1970.

1187. Gallager, D. W., et al. Dissociation between behavioral effects and changes in metabolism of cerebral serotonin (5HT) following Δ^9-tetrahydrocannabinol (THC). Pharmacologist 13:296, 1971.

1188. Menon, M. K., et al. Lowering of brain histamine (Hm) by parachlorophenylalanine (PSPA) and a new histidine decarboxylase inhibitor. Pharmacologist 12:205, 1970.

1189. Spaulding, T. C., et al. The pharmacological effects of and the lack of -THC blocking activity of phenitrone. Pharmacologist 13: 296, 1971.

1190. Hartmann, R. J. and I. Geller. Effects of para-chlorophenylalanine (p-CPA) on a conditioned emotional response (CER) in laboratory rats. Pharmacologist 12:206, 1970.

1191. Thompson, G. R., et al. Neurotoxicity of cannabinoids in chronically-treated rats and monkeys. Pharmacologist 13:296, 1971.

1192. Dewey, W. L., et al. Some acute and chronic interactions between Δ^9-THC and morphine in mice. Pharmacologist 13:296, 1971.

1193. Mantilla-Plata, B. and R. D. Harbison. Phenobarbital and SKF 525-A effect on Δ^9-tetrahydrocannabinol (THC) toxicity and distribution in mice. Pharmacologist 13:297, 1971.

1194. Gomoll, A. W., Comparative effects of propranolol (P) and sotalol (S) on myocardial contractility. Pharmacologist 12:213, 1970.

1195. Joy, R. M. and K. F. Killam. A comparison of acute and chronic diazepam on the EEG. Pharmacologist 12:218, 1970.

1196. Stern, W. C., et al. Effects of lysergic acid diethylamide (LSD) on sleep and spiking activity in the lateral geniculate nucleus (LGN) of the cat. Pharmacologist 13:306, 1971.

1197. Sawyer, N. and R. Mundy. Autonomic responses in the mouse. Pharmacologist 12: 246, 1970.

1198. Carlini, E. A., et al. Effects of (-) Δ^9-trans-tetrahydrocannabinol and a synthetic derivative on maze performance of rats. Pharmacology 4:359-368, 1970.

1199. Schlosser, W., et al. Indications of a possible dopamine reception at the spinal level. Pharmacologist 12:287, 1970.

1200. Spratto, G. R. and J. H. Mennear. Effects of propranolol on blood glucose responses in the mouse. Pharmacologist 11:253, 1969.

1201. Thut, P. D. and R. H. Rech. Electrocorticographic (ECoG) and behavioral effects of diethyldithiocarbamate (DDC) and L-DOPA. Pharmacologist 11:254, 1969.

1202. Barnes, C. D. and O. Pompeiano. The interaction of brain stem adrenergic systems and VIIIth nerve stimulation on the spinal cord. Neuropharmacol. 10:437-446, 1971.

1203. Bhattacharya, I. C. and L. Goldstein. Influence of acute and chronic nicotine administration on the electrical activity of the rabbit brain. Pharmacologist 11:254, 1969.

1204. Garrett, R. L. and J. H. Brown. Bradykinin-potentiated contractions induced by serotonin (5-HT), novepinephrine (NE) and potassium (K+) in rabbit aortic strips. Pharmacologist 12:347, 1970.

1205. Echols, S. D. and R. E. Jewett. Effects of morphine (M) on the sleep of cats. Pharmacologist 11:254, 1969.

BIBLIOGRAPHY

1206. Jaju, B. P. and S. C. Wang. Effects of diphenhydramine and dimenhydrinate on vestibular neuronal activity in cats. Pharmacologist 12:270, 1970.

1207. Peng, Tai-Chan and C. W. Cooper. The hypocalcenic effect of ethanol in rats and dogs. Pharmacologist 12:277, 1970.

1208. Chai, Kyoung and C. K. Erikson. Cholinergic modification of ethanol-induced EEG synchrony. Pharmacologist 12:277, 1970.

1209. Sharkawi, M. Effects of some centrally active drugs on acetylcholine synthesis in rat brain. Pharmacologist 12:294, 1970.

1210. Torchiana, M. L., et al. Pharmacological antagonism of the chronotropic and central manifestations of amitriptyline intoxication in unanesthetized dogs. Pharmacologist 11: 283, 1969.

1211. Gillis, R. A., et al. Effect of diphenylhydantoin on spontaneous sympathetic nerve activity. Pharmacologist 12:304, 1970.

1212. Arnold, A. and J. P. McAuliff. α-adrenergic receptor mediated hyperglycemia in the laboratory rodent. Pharmacologist 12: 306, 1970.

1213. Proudfit, H. K. and S. Norton. The effect of morphine on the evoked potential and multiunit activity of the rat superior colliculus. Fed. Proc. 29:252, 1970.

1214. Hazra, J. Disinhibition of the inhibitory effect of darkness on optic evoked potentials by lidocaine. Fed. Proc. 29:252, 1970.

1215. Goridis, C. and N. H. Neff. Monoamine oxidase: Approximation of turnover rates in brain and peripheral tissues of rat. Fed. Proc. 30:382, 1971.

1216. Cain, S. M. O_2 uptake during and after exercise with and without β-adrenergic blockade. Fed. Proc. 29:265, 1970.

1217. Thurman, A. E., et al. Altered vascular responsiveness-initial hypotensive mechanism of thiazide diuretics. Fed. Proc. 29:273, 1970.

1218. O'Rourke, R. A., et al. Effect of amyl nitrate and nitroglycerin on cardiovascular hemodynamics in the conscious animal. Fed. Proc. 29:274, 1970.

1219. Smith, C. M. and P. Luna. Effects of vasodilator drugs on ear skin temperatures in guinea pigs. Fed. Proc. 29:274, 1970.

1220. Vernadakis, A. and P. S. Timiras. Interrelation between convulsant drugs and X-radiation on the central nervous system of rats. Arch. int. Pharmacodyn. 170:146-151, 1967.

1221. Strobel, G. E. and H. Wollman. Pharmacology of anesthetic agents. Fed. Proc. 28: 1386-1403, 1969.

1222. Faingold, C. L. and C. A. Berry. Studies of antihistamine-induced EEG paroxysms in the cat. Fed. Proc. 29:384, 1970.

1223. Levin, P. The effect of anti-petit mal drugs on photic driving in the rabbit. Fed. Proc. 29:384, 1970.

1224. Dempsey, P. J., et al. Evidence for a direct myocardial effect of angiotensin. II. Fed. Proc. 29:389, 1970.

1225. Clark, C. and V. J. Lotti. Attenuation of the vomiting response to L-dopa after decarboxylase inhibition. Fed. Proc. 29:512, 1970.

1226. Tang, A. H. Effects of L-dopa on a polysynaptic spinal reflex of the rat. Fed. Proc. 29:512, 1970.

1227. Lomax, P. Animal pharmacology of marihuana. Proc. West. Pharmacol. Soc. 14:10-13, 1971.

1228. Koerpel, B. J. and L. D. Davis. Effect of lidocaine (L), propanolol (P) and MJ1999 on ouabain-induced changes in membrane potential of purkinje fibers. Fed. Proc. 29:517, 1970.

1229. Matsuzaki, M. and K. F. Killam. The effect of multiple doses of diphenylhydantoin on intensity discrimination in the cat. Proc. West. Pharmacol. Soc. 14:145-148, 1971.

1230. Uyeno, E. T. Behavioral effects of phenothiazines and barbiturates in the squirrel monkey. Proc. West. Pharmacol. Soc. 14: 149-153, 1971.

1231. Marchand, C., et al. The effect of SKF-525A on the distribution of CCl_4 in rats. Fed. Proc. 29:544, 1970.

1232. Clifford, D. H. and L. R. Soma. Feline anesthesia. Fed. Proc. 28:1479-1499, 1969.

1233. Weisenthal, L. Adrenergic mechanisms in relaxation of guinea pig taenia coli. Fed. Proc. 29:550, 1970.

1234. Weisse, A. B., et al. Prophylaxis and treatment of ventricular arrhythmias in acute myocardial infarction: A Comparison of three agents. Fed. Proc. 29:585, 1970.

1235. Hoar, R. M. Anesthesia in the guinea pig. Fed. Proc. 28:1517-1521, 1969.

1236. Cervoni, P. and E. Reit. Angiotensin and novepinephrine (NE): Interaction on the cat nictitating membrane. Fed. Proc. 29:614, 1970.

1237. Smith, A. A. and K. Hayashida. Blockade or reversal by propranolol of the narcotic and respiratory depression induced in mice by ethanol. Fed. Proc. 29:649, 1970.

1238. Dewey, W. L., et al. Some autonomic gastrointestinal and metabolic effects of two constituents of marihuana. Fed. Proc. 29: 650, 1970.

1239. Goldstein, M. L. Effect of LSD-25, and psilocybin on novepinephrine and 3H-novepinephrine metabolites in rat brain. Fed. Proc. 29:650, 1970.

1240. Goldstein, M., et al. The effects of antiparkinsonian drugs (AP) on striatal dopamine. Fed. Proc. 29:680, 1970.

1241. Kirkpatrick, W. E. and P. Lomax. Chlorpromazine and body temperature. Proc. West. Pharmacol. Soc. 13:169-172, 1970.

1242. Shaikh, M. I., et al. Acute and chronic effects of nicotine on rat gastric secretion. Proc. West. Pharmacol. Soc. 13:178-184, 1970.

1243. Tseng, L. F. and E. J. Walazek. Blockade of the dopamine response by bulbocapnine. Fed. Proc. 29:741, 1970.

1244. Lamarre, Y., et al. Harmaline-induced rhythmic activity of cerebellar and lower brain stem neurons. Brain Res. 32:246-250, 1971.

1245. Jondorf, W. R., et al. Inability of newborn mice and guinea pigs to metabolize drugs. Biochem. Pharmacol. 1:352-354, 1958.

1246. Davis, W. M. Day-night periodicity in pentobarbital response of mice and the influence of socio-psychological conditions. Experentia 18:235-237, 1962.

1247. Lutsky, I. Preoperative evaluation and preparation of canines. Fed. Proc. 28:1420-1422, 1969.

1248. Quinn, G. P., et al. Species, strain and sex differences in metabolism of hexabarbitone, amidopyrine, antipyrine and aniline. Biochem. Pharmacol. 1:152-159, 1958.

1249. Woods, L. A. and H. E. Muehlenbeck. Urinary excretion of codeine and its metabolite(s) in the day. J. Pharmacol. Exp. Ther. 110:54, 1954.

1250. Axelrod, J. Studies on sympathomimetic amines. I. The biotransformation and physiological disposition of l-norephedrine. J. Pharmacol. Exp. Ther. 109:62-73, 1953.

1251. Fuhrman, G. J. and F. A. Fuhrman. Effects of temperature on the action of drugs. Ann. Rev. Pharmacol. 1:65-78, 1961.

1252. Blair, E. Generalized hypothermia. Fed. Proc. 28:1456-1462, 1969.

1253. Goldstein, A., et al. Principles of drug action. The basis of pharmacology. Harper and Row, New York, 1968.

1254. Usubiaga, J. E., et al. Interaction of intravenously administered procaine, lidocaine and succinylcholine in anesthetized subjects. Anesth. and Analg. 46:39-45, 1967.

1255. Saidman, L. J. and E. I. Eger, II. The effect of thiopental metabolism on duration of anesthesia. Anesthesiology 27:118-126, 1966.

1256. Gillette, J. R., et al. Isolation from rat brain of a metabolic product, desmethylimipramine, that mediates the antidepressant activity of imipramine (Totranil). Experentia 17:417-418, 1961.

1257. Gillette, J. R. Biochemistry of drug oxidation and reduction by enzymes in hepatic endoplasmic reticulum. Adv. Pharmacol. 4: 219-261, 1966.

1258. Conney, A. Pharmacological implications of microsomal enzyme induction. Pharmacol. Rev. 19:317-366, 1967.

1259. Burns, J. J. and A. H. Conney. Enzyme stimulation and inhibition in the metabolism of drugs. Proc. Roy. Soc. Med. 58:955-960, 1965.

1260. Adams, H. R. and B. N. Dixit. Prolongation of pentobarbital anesthesia by chlorainphenical in dogs and cats. J.A.V.M.A. 156: 902-905, 1970.

1261. VanDyke, R. A. and M. B. Chenoweth. Metabolism of volatile anesthetics. Anesthesiology 26:348-357, 1965.

1262. VanDyke, R. A. Metabolism of volatile anesthetics, III. Induction of microsomal dechlorinating and ether-cleaving enzymes. J. Pharmacol. Exp. Ther. 154:364-369, 1966.

1263. Miller, E. V., et al. (Ed.) Comparative anesthesia in laboratory animals. Fed. Proc. 28:1373-1586, 1969.

1264. Priano, L. L., et al. Barbiturate anesthesia: An abnormal physiologic situation. J. Pharmacol. Exp. Ther. 165:126-135, 1969.

1265. VanCitters, R. L., et al. Left ventricular dynamics in dogs during anesthesia with α-chloralose and sodium pentobarbital. Am. J. Cardio. 13:349-354, 1964.

1266. Buss, B. G. and N. M. Buckley. Chloralose anesthesia in the dog: A study of drug actions and analytical methodology. Am. J. Physiol. 210:854-862, 1966.

1267. Maynert, E. W. The usefulness of clinical signs for the comparison of intravenous anesthetics in dogs. J. Pharmacol. Exp. Ther. 128:182-191, 1960.

1268. Maynert, E. W., et al. Acute tolerance to intravenous anesthetics in dogs. J. Pharmacol. Exp. Ther. 128:192-200, 1960.

1269. Wollman, H. and Dripps, R. D. Uptake, distribution, elimination and administration of inhalational anesthetics. In: The Pharmacological Basis of Therapeutics, Ed. Goodman and Gilman. 4th. edition, MacMillan Co., New York, 1970.

BIBLIOGRAPHY

1270. Stevens, W. C., et al. The cardiovascular effects of a new inhalation anesthetic, forane, in human volunteers at constant arterial carbon dioxide tension. Anesthesiology 35:8-16, 1971.

1271. Merkel, G. and E. Eger, II. A comparative study of halothane and halopropane anesthesia. Including method for determining equipotency. Anesthesiology 24:346-357, 1963.

1272. Waizer, P., et al. Microvascular reactions at known depth of anesthesia. Fed. Proc. 29: 354, 1970.

1273. Johnson, E. S., et al. The responses of cortical neurons to monoamines under differing anesthetic conditions. J. Physiol. 203: 261-280, 1969.

1274. Eger, E. I., II, et al. Temperature dependence of halothane and cyclopropane anesthesia in dogs: Correlation with some theories of anesthetic action. Anesthesiology 26:764-770, 1965.

1275. Eger, E. I., II., et al. Equipotent alveolar concentrations of methoxyflurane, halothane, diethyl ether, fluroxene, cyclopropane, xeron and nitrous oxide in the dog. Anesthesiology 26:771-777, 1965.

1276. Skorobogatov, V. I. The central action of curarizing drugs. In: Progress in Brain Research 20:243-255, 1967.

1277. Severinghaus, J. W. and C. P. Larson, Jr. Respiration in anesthesia. In: Fenn, W. O. and H. Rahn. Handbook of Physiology-Respiration II, 1219-1264, American Physiology Soc., Washington, D.C., 1965.

1278. Venes, J. L., et al. Nitrous oxide: an anesthetic for experiments in cats. Am. J. Physiol. 220:2028-2031, 1971.

INDEX

The following information is presented to illustrate the magnitude and scope of the index.

(1) <u>Indexing of Drug Names</u>: Each drug appearing in the main body of the handbook is indexed under its official name and, whenever possible, under three common names. For example, the pages where dosage information can be found for chlorpromazine are listed next to chlorpromazine, Largactil, Thorazine, and Megaphen.

(2) <u>Indexing of Drug Responses</u>: The page numbers, for each drug listed in the main body of the text, will also be found next to each pharmacological action that has been included for the particular drug. For example, the page numbers referring to chlorpromazine will appear next to: adrenolytic, analgetic, anticonvulsant, antiserotonin (<u>in vitro</u>), behavior, cardiovascular, electroencephalographic, hypothermic, Langendorff (<u>in vitro</u>), potentiate barbiturate sleep, rabbit (<u>in vitro</u>), sedative, sympatholytic.

mg/kg		Mouse	Rat	Guinea Pig	Rabbit	Cat	Dog	Monkey	
Lethal Dose $Y-LD_{50}$ $Z-MLD$	IV								
	IP								
	IM								
	SC								
	PO								
	IV								
	IP								
	IM								
	SC								
	PO								
	IV								
	IP								
	IM								
	SC								
	PO								
	IV								
	IP								
	IM								
	SC								
	PO								
	IV								
	IP								
	IM								
	SC								
	PO								
	IV								
	IP								
	IM								
	SC								
	PO								

mg/kg		Mouse	Rat	Guinea Pig	Rabbit	Cat	Dog	Monkey	
Lethal Dose $Y-LD_{50}$ $Z-MLD$	IV								
	IP								
	IM								
	SC								
	PO								
	IV								
	IP								
	IM								
	SC								
	PO								
	IV								
	IP								
	IM								
	SC								
	PO								
	IV								
	IP								
	IM								
	SC								
	PO								
	IV								
	IP								
	IM								
	SC								
	PO								
	IV								
	IP								
	IM								
	SC								
	PO								

mg/kg		Mouse	Rat	Guinea Pig	Rabbit	Cat	Dog	Monkey	
Lethal Dose $Y-LD_{50}$ $Z-MLD$	IV								
	IP								
	IM								
	SC								
	PO								
	IV								
	IP								
	IM								
	SC								
	PO								
	IV								
	IP								
	IM								
	SC								
	PO								
	IV								
	IP								
	IM								
	SC								
	PO								
	IV								
	IP								
	IM								
	SC								
	PO								
	IV								
	IP								
	IM								
	SC								
	PO								

mg/kg		Mouse	Rat	Guinea Pig	Rabbit	Cat	Dog	Monkey	
Lethal Dose $Y-LD_{50}$ $Z-MLD$	IV								
	IP								
	IM								
	SC								
	PO								
	IV								
	IP								
	IM								
	SC								
	PO								
	IV								
	IP								
	IM								
	SC								
	PO								
	IV								
	IP								
	IM								
	SC								
	PO								

IN VITRO

mg %	Cardiac	Vascular	Gut	Uterine	Visceral	Skeletal		

mg/kg		Mouse	Rat	Guinea Pig	Rabbit	Cat	Dog	Monkey	
Lethal Dose $Y-LD_{50}$ $Z-MLD$	IV								
	IP								
	IM								
	SC								
	PO								
	IV								
	IP								
	IM								
	SC								
	PO								
	IV								
	IP								
	IM								
	SC								
	PO								
	IV								
	IP								
	IM								
	SC								
	PO								

IN VITRO

mg %	Cardiac	Vascular	Gut	Uterine	Visceral	Skeletal		

mg/kg		Mouse	Rat	Guinea Pig	Rabbit	Cat	Dog	Monkey	
Lethal Dose $Y-LD_{50}$ $Z-MLD$	IV								
	IP								
	IM								
	SC								
	PO								
	IV								
	IP								
	IM								
	SC								
	PO								
	IV								
	IP								
	IM								
	SC								
	PO								
	IV								
	IP								
	IM								
	SC								
	PO								

IN VITRO

mg %	Cardiac	Vascular	Gut	Uterine	Visceral	Skeletal		